YOGA
to the RESCUE
Ageless Beauty

How to Keep Yourself Glowingly
Beautiful Inside and Out!

AMY LUWIS

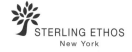

STERLING ETHOS
New York

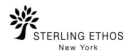

STERLING ETHOS
New York

An Imprint of Sterling Publishing
387 Park Avenue South
New York, NY 10016

STERLING ETHOS and the distinctive Sterling logo are
registered trademarks of Sterling Publishing Co., Inc.

© 2012 by Amy Luwis

All rights reserved. No part of this publication may be reproduced, stored in a retrieval system,
or transmitted, in any form or by any means, electronic, mechanical, photocopying, recording,
or otherwise, without prior written permission from the publisher.

ISBN 978-1-4027-8415-6 (paperback)
ISBN 978-1-4549-0255-3 (ebook)

Distributed in Canada by Sterling Publishing
c/o Canadian Manda Group, 165 Dufferin Street
Toronto, Ontario, Canada M6K 3H6
Distributed in the United Kingdom by GMC Distribution Services
Castle Place, 166 High Street, Lewes, East Sussex, England BN7 1XU
Distributed in Australia by Capricorn Link (Australia) Pty. Ltd.
P.O. Box 704, Windsor, NSW 2756, Australia

For information about custom editions, special sales, and premium and corporate purchases,
please contact Sterling Special Sales at 800-805-5489 or specialsales@sterlingpublishing.com.

Manufactured in China

2 4 6 8 10 9 7 5 3 1

www.sterlingpublishing.com

Buying from breeders leads to the needless death of millions of dogs and cats each year. I dedicate this book with all my heart to everyone who adopts and works toward ending this tragedy.

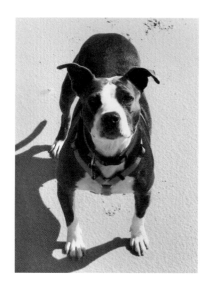

My beloved Rescued pit bull, Isabelle.
Pit bulls are the sweetest dogs in the world.
Adopted from the amazing
rescue group BullyPaws.org.

"Until one has loved an animal, a part of one's soul remains unawakened."

—Anatole France

This book is not intended to diagnose, treat, cure, or prevent any disease or condition. If you have a health concern or condition, consult your doctor or health care provider. Always consult your doctor before starting any new exercise program.

Contents

Prologue

I'm a voracious reader of self-improvement books. At the moment, I have a stack of books next to my bed that, if toppled, could do some serious damage to my nose. I'm also a bit obsessive about researching and procuring new things from around the globe that will make me look and feel better and help me live an incredibly long time; I'm so passionate about all of this that I've lured my family into my lair of elixirs and regimes. My biggest target (besides myself) is my beloved mother who—to her amazing credit—is always game for trying something new.

One of the biggest challenges I face is the voluminous amount of conflicting material I come across and knowing how to process it all. One minute I read that coffee is good for me, the next minute I read it will put me into an early grave. I've come to the ultimate conclusion that there are a tiny handful of absolute truths, like that smoking is very, very, very bad for you and that exercise is very, very, very good for you, and that you should eat lots and lots of colorful vegetables. The rest fall somewhere in between.

The majority of health books that I read contain top-notch advice on wellness, but my issue is that they're just plain overwhelming. They are packed with an infinite amount of suggestions, from supplements to regimes that would demand the dedication of a monk. Not only is this unrealistic, it is highly impractical and somewhat loony—we're already so overwhelmed in our daily lives!

I am also someone who is unabashedly on the lazy end of the spectrum. I believe that anything worthwhile or lasting shouldn't be tedious and, to me, a day overflowing with regimes and supplements pretty much equals torture. So, I weed through and pluck what I believe to be the superstars of healthy living and attempt to incorporate them into my week. My list does not contain fads or fleeting ideas. On the contrary, it contains wonderful, youth-enhancing elements, some of which have been around for centuries and are exceptionally helpful.

Before I share this amazingly wonderful list with you, I have a confession to make. True, I love yoga and am constantly adding healthy bits to my life, but I also have a "dark side" (don't we all?) and I call her ToxicGirl. ToxicGirl is mischievous, disobedient, disorderly, and unruly. She stays up super-late eating cake and she washes it down with a bottle of champagne. She has a wicked temper, loves to hold grudges, Googles ex-beaus and ex-friends, and shops online way too much.

I've tried to leave her behind many times and reside in my temple of perfection—living the purest of pure lives—but she always finds her way back in the door. Now that I'm older, I'm done trying to get rid of her; in fact, I'm learning to accept her, and when I do, she seems to behave herself better. You see, I think life is messy and it is not meant to be perfect, nor are we supposed to be perfect in it. I think we are simply here to do our best and accept ourselves exactly as we are. So there you go, I'm not always doing yoga; sometimes I'm stuffing my face with cake. I'm not always incorporating every single thing on my list, because I'm too busy shopping online and drinking champagne! And at this very moment as I write this prologue, it is 10:30 a.m., I'm still in my pajamas, and I'm eating chocolate and licorice.

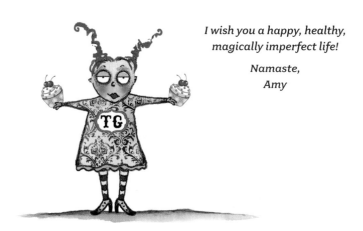

I wish you a happy, healthy, magically imperfect life!

Namaste,
Amy

Amy's Superstar Health List

Magical tips to keep you glowing on the inside and outside

. . . .

Inversions

Has your skin lost its glow?

Then do some inversions to erase those wrinkles and give yourself radiant skin. Inversions also saturate your brain with oxygen-rich blood, flooding it with essential nutrients (your eyes, facial capillaries, and hair will receive more oxygen and nutrients in the process, too!).

Inversions boost lymphatic drainage* and detoxification, reducing cellulite, acne, and varicose veins. Inversions will also improve your memory and concentration, not just make your skin look great! They also improve posture (no one with poor posture ever looks youthful!).

Inversions can be intimidating and challenging, so try an easy and amazingly beneficial one called Legs-Up-the-Wall Pose (see *Ageless* category). Do this every day, and watch the years melt away (yogis call this pose the fountain of youth).

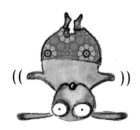

* What the heck is lymphatic drainage and why should I care? The lymphatic system plays an important role in the body's immune functions and is your first line of defense against disease. This vast network transports and filters lymph fluid, which contains a jumble of stuff from the good (antibodies) to the bad (toxins); not only does it filter out toxins, but it regenerates tissue, restores hydration of the skin, minimizes lines and wrinkles, relieves chronic pain, and oh, so much more!

When the lymphatic system is blocked and lymph fluid stagnates, all havoc can break loose, so stimulating this system to get that fluid flowing and draining is essential.

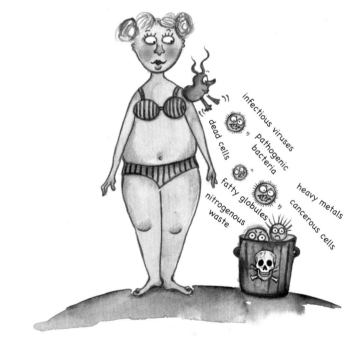

infectious viruses

dead cells

pathogenic bacteria

heavy metals

fatty globules

cancerous cells

nitrogenous waste

Thoughts Are Things

Just like cupcakes and flowers, thoughts are "solid," not just some ephemeral bits floating in the recesses of our brains. There is an explosion of recent material on this subject, from the movie *The Secret* to Candace B. Pert's book *Molecules of Emotion: The Science Behind Mind-Body Medicine*, but "law of attraction" goes much farther back than this. I think transcendentalist Henry David Thoreau said it best in his classic book, *Walden*: "I learned this, at least, by my experiment; that if one advances confidently in the direction of his dreams, and endeavors to live the life which he has imagined, he will meet with a success unexpected in common hours. He will put some things behind, will pass an invisible boundary; new, universal, and more liberal laws will begin to establish themselves around and within him; or the old laws will be expanded, and interpreted in his favor in a more liberal sense, and he will live with the license of a higher order of beings."

So be mindful of your thoughts throughout the day and practice switching off the negative thoughts and replacing them with positive, happy thoughts! The more you do this, the more wonderful things and people will come into your life.

Sleep
Don't skimp on it

While you sleep, your body is busily producing 80 percent of your growth hormones. Why should you care? Because these precious hormones slow down the aging process and heal and repair things in your body, as an excellent mechanic would.

If someone said to you, "There is one simple thing you can do that will help regulate your weight, increase your energy, productivity, and mental clarity, and improve your emotions." Would you jump on board? If the answer is an enthusiastic "yes," then

"It is a common experience that a problem difficult at night is resolved in the morning after the committee of sleep has worked on it." —John Steinbeck

all you have to do is follow Benjamin Franklin's advice, written over two hundred years ago: *"Early to bed, and early to rise, makes a man healthy, wealthy, and wise."*

The earlier you get to sleep, the better. Before 10 p.m. would be magnificent, but 11 p.m. will do in order to reap the benefits. The amount of sleep needed varies from person to person. I find that I need a full eight hours of sleep.

Hot Water*
A nice little weight-loss friend

Sip hot water throughout the day and you will lose weight. I repeat, you will lose weight. (Sharon's Story, page 93, *The Ageless Woman* by Nancy Lonsdorf, MD).

The ideal hot water program: Boil some pure water (spring, filtered, etc.) for at least 10 minutes—boil enough water, so you can sip it throughout the day (I usually boil about 4 cups of water). Boiling it for this long energizes the water. When water boils, it becomes sharper and more therapeutic, which allows it to cleanse the body's channels (the channels of your body—for example, the intestines and kidneys—carry nutrients to the cells and carry waste out of the body); when your channels are cleansed it makes it easier for water to hydrate the tissues and removes toxins and impurities from your system. Boiled water also optimizes digestion and metabolism and reduces cravings!

Put your water in a large thermos and take a few sips every half hour throughout the day until 8 p.m.

Also, sipping a small amount of hot water during a meal is good, but don't drink too much of any liquid with your meals, because it dilutes your digestive juices, making it harder to digest food!

*If you have high blood pressure, please consult your doctor before embarking on this regime.

Water and Weight-Loss

Drinking water may be the most important piece to the weight-loss puzzle. Water contains no calories, fat, or cholesterol and is low in sodium. It is nature's appetite-suppressant, and it helps the body to metabolize fat. Current research shows that low water intakes yield an increase in fat deposits. Conversely, a high water intake reduces the amount of fat deposits. Without enough water, the kidneys cannot function properly. As a result, some of their workload is pushed off on to the liver, in turn preventing the liver from operating at peak levels.

How does all this tie into weight loss? Because metabolizing fat is a primary function of the liver, and because the liver can't function at peak levels when taking on the added workload from the kidneys, less body fat is metabolized and more is stored. This leads to either weight gain or reaching a plateau of weight loss. Dieting typically involves restricting the number of calories taken in, which usually involves lessening the total amount of water available to the body, since about 30 percent of the average person's water intake comes from food. So, dieting is an important time to raise your water intake.

Dry Brushing

Skin brushing is a simple way to beautify and cleanse the body. Daily brushing improves circulation, stimulates the lymphatic system (the system responsible for eliminating toxins), reduces the appearance of cellulite, exfoliates dry skin, and encourages new cell growth . . . yahoo!

After a few years of hearing about the miracles of dry brushing, I finally bought myself a sisal body brush (made in Japan, costs around eight dollars, and is a nice-quality brush). Keep in mind, unless you get a brush with a handle or enlist your partner, reaching your whole back will take some very limber arms. At first, I thought I was just imagining all the great benefits, but after thirty days of dry brushing every morning, I'm a true believer in this prickly accessory! Brushing my body is like brushing my teeth now—I never miss a day (well, almost); it energizes me, makes my skin velvety soft, my leg hair grows more slowly and comes in softer, *and* the best thing, my jiggly bits are a bit firmer! I now refer to my sisal brush as my magic wand and I travel with it.

Dry Brushing 101

"Dry" brush your body—most people are in the habit of wetting down a brush in the shower then scrubbing, which defeats the purpose of dry brushing! I've bought my mom several brushes, she promises to keep them away from water and keep them dryer than straw, and then I see the brushes damp and hanging in her shower—blasphemy!

It's an economical spa treatment—as noted, you can get a good quality body brush for under ten dollars. Dry brush in the morning before getting dressed. It will energize you better than a cup of coffee.

Tea

Boost your immunity and antioxidant levels by drinking white or green tea

White tea is made from baby tea leaves and is processed less than green tea and has much less caffeine. Because it remains much closer to its natural state than green tea, it contains many more polyphenols—the powerful antioxidants that hunt down and kill cancer-causing cells.

Need another reason to drink white tea? A 2004 study* found that white tea is pretty darn good at fighting off viruses and dangerous, infection-causing bacteria. So think about switching that latté to white tea or, at the very least, adding a few cups to your diet every day!

Green tea rocks, too! Especially matcha (a finely milled green tea or powdered green tea), because you ingest the whole tea leaf, not just the brewed water from the tea leaf. What does that translate to? The antioxidant and nutritional benefits you get from drinking ten cups of regular green tea can be found in a single cup of matcha! This will save you many trips to the bathroom, and according to Dr. Andrew Weil, will give you a feeling of well-being.

Coffee

Think moderation

Seriously consider replacing coffee (both regular and decaffeinated) with white tea, green tea, Rooibos tea, or Raja's Cup (a traditional Ayurvedic beverage that promotes well-being and vitality, stimulates the mind, is a powerful antioxidant, diminishes stress, and eliminates toxins). This fabulous coffee substitute is a blend of four potent herbs—clearing nut, kasmard, licorice, and winter cherry. Don't want to replace your beloved cup of coffee? (I don't, but I limit myself to one to two cups on the weekends while perusing a good book.) Then simply add the above to your weekly liquid intake or better yet, replace a few cups of java with some healthy tea!

*Science*Daily (May 28, 2004)

Sugar
(Satan in a little white suit)

At the risk of sounding a bit dramatic, sugar is a socially acceptable, celebrated, legal recreational drug and just like other harmful drugs, it destroys your health over time. Here are just a few of the things regular consumption of sugar can do to your body and mind: disrupt normal brain function; produce a significant rise in total cholesterol, triglycerides, and bad cholesterol (LDL); decrease good cholesterol (HDL); directly cause diabetes and obesity; drain the body of vitamins and minerals; weaken the immune system, and cause a loss of tissue elasticity and function. . . . This list goes on and could fill a book, so avoiding or limiting this seductive sweet would be a very wise decision.

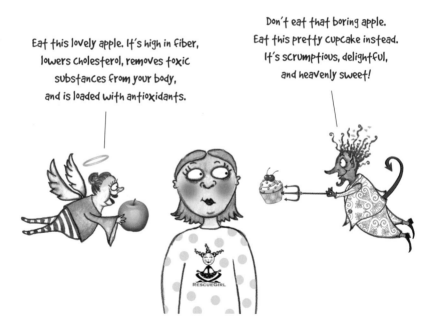

Eat this lovely apple. It's high in fiber, lowers cholesterol, removes toxic substances from your body, and is loaded with antioxidants.

Don't eat that boring apple. Eat this pretty cupcake instead. It's scrumptious, delightful, and heavenly sweet!

RESCUEGIRL

Before you start mourning the loss of your dear friends Mademoiselle Cupcake and Monsieur Moon Pie, know that there are excellent healthy alternative sweeteners on the market today: Agave nectar, known as "honey water" in Mexico, used for thousands of years and prized by the Aztecs as a gift from the gods, is so delicious, you'll forget that sugar ever existed.

Unlike the empty calorie, life-zapping properties of sugar, agave actually has major health benefits! Agave contains saponins and fructans; these are anti-inflammatory and boost immunity. Also, compared to other sweeteners, agave has a very desirable low-glycemic index, which means it won't cause a sharp rise or fall in blood sugar.

Stevia is another healthy alternative sweetener to sugar without sugar's unhealthy drawbacks. Stevia is an herb that grows wild as a small shrub in South America, and it's been used throughout the world as a sugar substitute and medicinal aid for centuries. Stevia contains phytonutrients, minerals, and vitamins and it's known to stabilize blood sugar levels.

If you're craving a sweet, try one of my favorite snacks—dried Medjool dates with a dab of peanut butter. This remarkable little fruit is not only amazingly sweet, it is loaded with potassium (just one little date has more potassium than a banana), packed with dietary fiber, and contains vital amino acids that aid digestion.

Lemon* Water
Start your day with it

Traditional Chinese Medicine suggests waking your body up gently in the morning with a glass of warm lemon water, this not only hydrates your body when you first wake up, but it also rids your body of toxins that have built up in your system overnight.

---

*Lemon tip: Lemons should be kept at room temperature. To extract the most juice and pulp, roll the lemon on a counter with the palm of your hand to break up the membranes that hold the juice (this makes it so much easier to juice the lemon).

Seaweed

Think like a mermaid!

One of a few magical superfoods, not only is seaweed superior in nutrition to land vegetables, but it's also a great little helper for losing weight.

Sea vegetables are much higher in important minerals and trace elements than land vegetables. Phytochemicals found only in sea vegetables cleanse the body of nasty pollutants. Radioactive elements and heavy metals such as mercury bind with seaweed's alginic acid in the intestines, render them indigestible, and then eliminate them from your body. How's that for a deep cleanse!

Sea vegetables are also an excellent source of protein, fiber, enzymes, and vitamins.

And that's not all! Sea vegetables have also been proven to help reverse cardiovascular disease, shrink tumors, promote weight-loss by stimulating the thyroid, boost the immune system, and decrease blood sugar.

Some types of seaweeds are: nori, kombu, wakame, bladderwrack, and arame. Arame is the mildest tasting of the sea vegetables.

If you'd rather lick a sidewalk than eat fresh seaweed, then consider incorporating a seaweed extract or seaweed pills from a reputable company that certifies that their products are pure*. An excellent place to start: www.seaveg.com. They carry sustainably harvested and certified organic edible seaweed, and it is delicious! Give it a try, you may be surprised how much you like it.

*Fresh, dried, extracts, pills: No matter what form of seaweed you prefer, always purchase from a reputable company since seaweed can be easily contaminated with toxic substances.

Reishi

A mushroom a day keeps the doctor away

I stumbled upon an amazing website a few years ago called Fungi Perfecti (www.fungi.com) and learned things I never knew about the world of mushrooms. I no longer saw these shy little creatures as a nice accent to my soup, but as little miracles of nature. Fungi Perfecti was founded by mycologist, environmentalist, and author Paul Stamets. The man truly knows his mushrooms, so I read up on reishi, and a love affair was born.

Reishi is one of the big stars of the mushroom world and a particular favorite of mine. The reishi mushroom is known as the "king of herbs" in Traditional Chinese Medicine, and classical literature refers to it as a "superior herb." It has been used for over 2,000 years and is a safe, nontoxic herb. It's ability to regulate and fine-tune the immune system is legendary, and it also reduces inflammation, increases blood flow, and has strong antioxidant properties.

Reishi mushrooms are believed to suppress tumor growth and are often used in cancer prevention efforts for this reason.

There are various varieties of reishi, but the most effective in improving overall health is red reishi, which can be found in tincture or tablet form. It is also available dry and can be ground in a coffee grinder and made into a tea that has a bitter edge (which I actually like). You can also add it to things like soup stock.

After reading up on reishi, you may want to incorporate this mushroom into your daily diet.

Vegetables
Think like a rabbit

Like many people, I grew up on a steady diet of meat, and it never occurred to me that the stuff I was eating came from an animal just like my beloved cat, Cinders, whose belly I'd rub while dousing my meatloaf with ketchup. Oh, the irony! When I was twenty-two I read a book that changed my life, *Animal Liberation* by Peter Singer. It's a quick read with a very profound message that turned me into a die-hard vegetarian.

I was quite radical when I was younger, yelling at and alienating friends and family who allowed a brisket or burger to pass through their lips. But now that I'm older, I've mellowed, and am tickled pink by meat-eaters who at least make an effort: adding a few meat-free days a week, buying certified-humane animal products, boycotting the cruelest—foie gras and veal, for example. Of course, I'd prefer that the world go vegetarian, but I gave up on this pipe dream years ago, realizing that many people want what they want—even if it means an animal must suffer enormously.

No matter how you slice it, a meat-based diet isn't good for your body, your soul, or the planet, and if you're not convinced of any of this, then check out the eye opening and entertaining films *Food, Inc.*, *Fast Food Nation*, and *Supersize Me* and the brilliant and captivating books *Animal Liberation* by Peter Singer and *The Omnivore's Dilemma* by Michael Pollan.

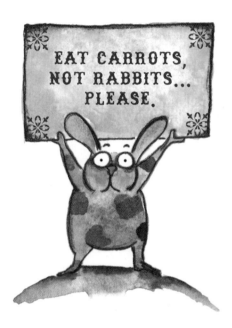

"A human being is a part of a whole, called by us 'universe,' a part limited in time and space. He experiences himself, his thoughts and feelings as something separated from the rest . . . a kind of optical delusion of his consciousness. This delusion is a kind of prison for us, restricting us to our personal desires and to affection for a few persons nearest to us. Our task must be to free ourselves from this prison by widening our circle of compassion to embrace all living creatures and the whole of nature in its beauty."

—Albert Einstein

Introduction

How to make your yoga practice extra fabulous!

....

The Beauty of Yoga

In a world filled with uncertainty and clashing views, it's a refreshingly indisputable fact that yoga not only helps heal the body, but also prevents disease. It's also one of the best ways to ensure a youthful body and mind at any age.

Practicing yoga on a regular basis will give you a strong, flexible body, supple spine, and excellent posture. It will unclutter your mind, calm your nerves, and give you a more joyful outlook on life. It's also pretty darn good at reducing cellulite.

You don't have to maintain a rigorous practice either, just ten to twenty minutes a day will bring you amazing benefits. It is more important to be consistent and do a little most days than to cram in a long session once a week.

Another great perk? Yoga is simple and it's unique to every individual. There is no such thing as the "perfect" pose. Any pose can be modified to meet your needs and challenges. It doesn't matter if you are eight or eighty, flexible or stiff as a board, clumsy or graceful, yoga will work its magic on you, you simply need to practice consistently a little bit each day. A few poses in front of the TV is better than no yoga at all.

Pranayama (breath control) is the cornerstone of yoga: Proper breathing will invigorate and

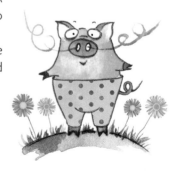

ALWAYS BREATHE THROUGH YOUR NOSE—
THIS FILTERS AND WARMS THE AIR BEFORE
IT ENTERS YOUR BEAUTIFUL BODY!

enliven your yoga practice. On the contrary, *poor* breathing will dull and stagnate it. So remember to *breeeeeeeeeeathe!*

Breathing Tips and Pointers

Always breathe through your nose, which filters and warms the air before it enters your body.

Breathe evenly, steadily, and deeply, not forcefully, and focus on expanding your belly first, then your chest.

Your breath should flow consistently and easily while doing yoga poses. If you find yourself holding your breath or if you are breathing unevenly or strenuously, then this is a good indicator that you probably need to ease up or modify the pose.

Let your intuition guide your breathing, while keeping these simple guidelines in mind: Exhale when moving into a pose, folding your body, and when starting or deepening a twist. Inhale when coming out of a pose, expanding your chest, and when you extend your body up or out.

Be Mindful

Being present in the moment and in your body while practicing poses will deepen your yoga practice. Focusing on your breath will help keep you in the moment and silence the endless chatter in your head—think proper alignment, breathing, and balance, *not* unpaid bills, deadlines, and dirty laundry!

Take inventory like a stockroom employee, from your head to your toes: *What hurts? What feels good? Is my mind quiet or distracted? Am I properly aligned? Is something out of balance? Am I putting emphasis on the wrong body part?* If something hurts, modify your position or stop all together. If you feel good, try deepening the pose. If your mind is scattered and distracted, focus on your breathing.

Strike a pose: Beginners should hold poses for three to five breath cycles (one cycle is one inhalation and one exhalation). You can increase this as you feel comfortable.

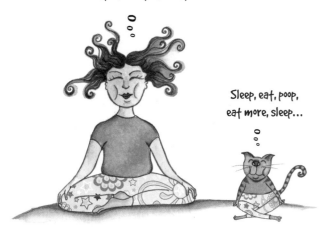

Be a unique yogini: You don't need to do any pose exactly like the illustration shows, just simply find the right place within the pose that's perfect for you (hint: it should not feel painful!) and progress more deeply into a pose as your body allows.

If you find yourself losing your balance and falling out of a pose, don't worry. Be confident and say to yourself, "I'm graceful, strong, and perfect exactly as I am." Then try the pose again.

Pain is not gain: If you feel pain, stop what you are doing. Challenge yourself, but don't push yourself to a point of pain or discomfort. After all, yoga should be fun and uplifting, or else you won't do it!

Think like a tortoise: Don't blast through yoga poses. Do them mindfully, gently, and slowly.

Secrets of sequencing: Opposite poses attract. For example, after doing Downward Facing Dog, do Upward Facing Dog. After expanding your body in Bow Pose, contract your body in Boat Pose! A twist to the right balances with a twist to the left. Always do both sides of asymmetrical poses.

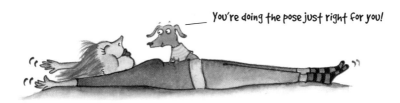
You're doing the pose just right for you!

In general, a yoga sequence should have a beginning, a middle, and an end. Start by waking up the body, progress into a few challenging poses, and always end a sequence with a restorative, calming pose like Downward Facing Corpse Pose.

That time of the month: During your period avoid standing poses, invigorating poses like back bends, and inversions; these can overtax your system and mess up the natural rhythm of your cycle. But by all means do seated forward bends, seated poses, and twists; all of these provide relief—relief from cramps, headache, fatigue, swelling, lower back pain, and more.

Tips for Newbies

- Without even realizing it, most people tend to tense up in the neck and shoulders, so be aware of this when doing poses and stay relaxed.

- Choose easier poses (an obvious, but often overlooked suggestion).

- Rest between poses.

- Move into and out of poses slowly.

- Breathe evenly and steadily, and don't hold your breath.

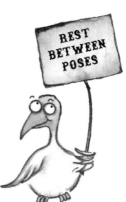

REST BETWEEN POSES

- Hold a pose for a shorter period of time and repeat it a few times, rather than holding it longer.

- Use props; straps, blocks, bolsters, and blankets can reduce the difficulty of a pose and make it easier for you to attempt more advanced poses, too.

Mini-Yoga is Better than No-Yoga!

- Do Raised Arms Pose (see *Joy* category) while waiting in line at the grocery store. Do it without the raised arms if you're a bit shy. Imagine the crown of your head being pulled up by a string, like you're a puppet; feel your spine lift and elongate. Imagine your feet anchored to the floor. This is an excellent way to practice good posture.

- Stuck in a traffic jam? Take a few deep belly breaths, center yourself on your sit bones, and do some shoulder rolls.

- Need an energy boost at the office? Do a modified Sage Twist (see *Pain* category). Sit sideways on an armless chair, center yourself on your sit bones, and anchor yourself to the ground. Elongate your spine (poor posture significantly limits your spinal rotation), bring your awareness to your lower back, and begin the twist from there. Let the twist gradually move up your spine (don't twist quickly), and with each exhalation, deepen the twist a little bit more. Release slowly.

- Need a quick stress reliever? Do one of my favorite daily poses, Standing Forward Bend (see *Ageless* category), for a minute.

- For the ultimate in rejuvenation (in a hotel, office, or at home), try Crocodile or Downward Facing Corpse Pose (see *Serenity* category).

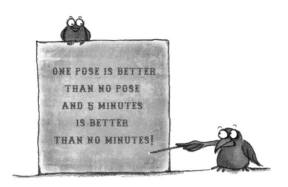

ONE POSE IS BETTER
THAN NO POSE
AND 5 MINUTES
IS BETTER
THAN NO MINUTES!

A Cornucopia of Poses

Standing poses: Standing poses should form the core of a beginner's yoga practice. They establish a strong foundation, invigorate and strengthen the whole body, and enhance stability and balance. (All standing poses stem from Mountain Pose.)

Your legs provide the base of support in standing poses. Make this base strong by anchoring your feet into the ground—weight evenly distributed, legs engaged and strong—and align your body. Do this, and you'll be well equipped to meet the challenges of standing poses and reap their many amazing benefits!

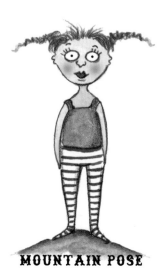

MOUNTAIN POSE

Forward bends and backbends: Forward bends are excellent poses to encourage going inward and deep reflection. They also soothe the nervous system and have a calming effect. Forward bends are also good for stimulating the internal organs, so you can digest food more easily and remove toxins from your body.

In daily life there is an abundance of bending forward—you bend forward to wash dishes, tie your shoes, and drive a car; and you probably spend hours hunched in front of a computer. Most people rarely find the occasion to bend backward, but backbends are magnificent for improving your mood, opening your chest, and expanding your lungs, allowing more oxygen to flow in. They enliven your spine, which in turn enlivens your whole body!

Don't force your body into these poses. Take your time and only move into a pose as far as you can comfortably. Deepening these poses comes as a result of relaxing into them, letting go of all tension. Straining to go further into a bend puts excessive pressure on the spine, so maintain a constant awareness of your spine and be gentle with it.

A twist a day: Twists detoxify your organs, improve your circulation, and help restore your spine's range of motion. When you release a twist, your organs get flooded with nutrients, and toxins are released. Twists are also excellent for improving digestion and releasing tension.

Twists are extremely beneficial for women; twists rejuvenate, tone, and massage the reproductive organs.

The trick to garnering the most benefits from twists is to do them correctly and for the right length of time, so heed these golden rules: (1) Make sure you have a strong foundation and you are anchored firmly into the ground. (2) Start with an elongated spine as you move into the twist. (3) As with all poses, the deeper effects of a twist are experienced when you hold it longer (at least a minute, and longer is even better).

Bonus! Let your eyes twist along with your spine. When focusing and stretching your eye muscles, you clear away toxins, tone the area around the eyes, and diminish wrinkles.

Inversions: These poses can be more challenging than other poses, but they're well worth it.

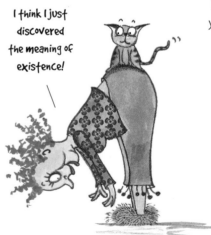

I think I just discovered the meaning of existence!

Unless you work for Cirque de Soleil, you probably spend the majority of your day with your head *above* your heart and your hips and legs *below* your heart. When you do an inversion (putting your brain below your heart) the body and mind reap all sorts of spectacular benefits. Inversions reverse the aging effect of gravity; bring emotional balance and mental clarity; improve blood flow to and from the heart; help regulate blood pressure, glucose levels, and chemical balance; boost brain power (blood flow to the brain is increased, nourishing the brain cells with more oxygen and nutrients required for optimal brain function); strengthen the immune system; improve lymph and blood circulation; relieve fatigue and depression.

Blood flow to the brain gradually decreases with age, and senility can set in; inversions increase circulation to the upper body, increasing blood to the brain, without putting strain on the heart.

In a nutshell, inversions turn gravity upside down and are therefore among the best means of slowing down and even reversing the aging process!

Consider doing Legs-Up-the-Wall Pose every day.

Restorative poses are deceptively simple, but require awareness and practice; they should be a part of every yoga routine, and every sequence should end with one. They are an excellent way to renew and heal after a stressful day.

Here are a few things to remember when performing a restorative pose: (1) Keep your props handy—blankets, blocks, straps, towel, eye bag, pillows, etc.— because they will help support your body and allow you to sink deeper into the pose. (2) Take plenty of time to get comfortable in the pose, tweaking and adjusting your props until you feel blissfully comfortable. You will be surprised what a tiny tweak of a rolled towel can do for your neck! (3) Above all else, let your intuition be your guide.

Last, but not least: Enjoy this book. Hold on to the bits that work for you and inspire you, and ignore the rest!

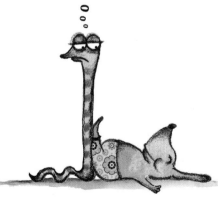

She needs to learn the difference between a wall and a snake.

Ageless

Do you want to look and feel young no matter what age you are? Then throw out those negative thoughts, give worrying the boot, lead with a loving heart, and practice yoga!

There isn't one simple answer to something as complex as aging, but there is one simple fact: practicing yoga* turns back the clock and slows down the aging process—as little as ten to twenty minutes a day will improve your physical appearance and mental acuity—your skin will glow, your posture will improve, and you'll remember where you left your keys!

*Relaxing your face is an important part of yoga and is fundamental to de-stressing: the muscles in your face are all connected to other parts of your body. When your face is tense it usually means you're holding a lot of tension in the rest of your body. So, relaxing your face, from your forehead to your jaw, will not only help smooth out those wrinkles, it will relax your entire body!

Lion Pose
(Simhasana)

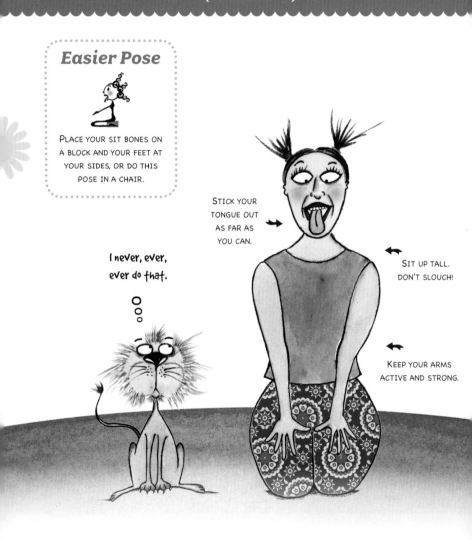

Easier Pose

PLACE YOUR SIT BONES ON A BLOCK AND YOUR FEET AT YOUR SIDES, OR DO THIS POSE IN A CHAIR.

STICK YOUR TONGUE OUT AS FAR AS YOU CAN.

SIT UP TALL. DON'T SLOUCH!

KEEP YOUR ARMS ACTIVE AND STRONG.

I never, ever, ever do that.

Wobbly neck?

This stimulates the platysma (a muscle on the front of the throat) and keeps it firm as you age.

1. Kneel on the floor, knees shoulder-width apart, top of feet flat on the floor.

2. Sit back on your heels (the front of your legs should be flat on the floor).

3. Rest your hands on your knees, fingers spread apart.

4. Move your knees a little farther apart.

5. Roll your shoulders back and sit up tall.

6. While maintaining a straight spine, lean forward slightly.

7. Open your mouth and eyes wide and stick your tongue out and down.

8. Gaze at the tip of your nose.

9. Lift your arms off your knees slightly (keep your fingers spread).

10. Hold for a few seconds.

11. Relax.

    Repeat 3 times.

Benefits

Eases tension in the face and jaw (excellent for TMJ/jaw clenchers!); relieves a sore throat; increases courage; boosts mood; traditional texts say that *Simhasana* eliminates disease.

Focus Points & Tips

Keep your spine long; keep your neck and shoulders relaxed; roar like a lion to stimulate the throat and increase courage.

Ouch   If you have knee issues, use caution when performing flexed-knee sitting positions.

Eye Rejuvenation

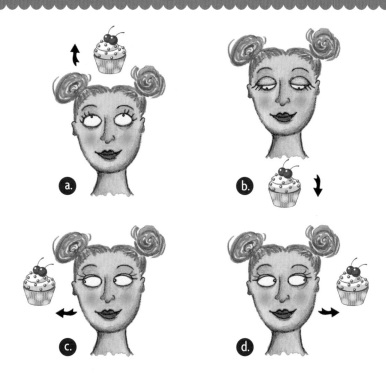

Eyesight is very precious, yet many people think more about exercising their derriere than their eyes! Eye muscles can weaken with age and become stiff and rigid—like any muscle in the body that doesn't get exercise—resulting in vision problems. Loss of elasticity reduces the ability of the lens of the eye to focus at different distances; eyesight also becomes weaker. Eye tension is also very common today because of long hours spent in front of glowing screens, from computers to cell phones and other mobile devices (eye tension stresses the brain and can cause overall tension and anxiety). So exercise those beautiful eyes!

1 Lie down on a yoga mat or a few folded blankets or sit in a firm chair in a comfortable position with your hands on your knees (don't slouch!).

2 Without straining your eyes or moving your head—look up as high as you can at a fixed point (a.), then look down as low as you can at a fixed point (b.). Repeat 3 times, then release and blink quickly a few times.

3 Without straining your eyes or moving your head—look to the right as far as you can at a fixed point (c.), then look to the left as far as you can at a fixed point (d.). Repeat 3 times, then release and blink quickly a few times.

(continued on page 29)

Keep your eyes gorgeous

Drink plenty of water throughout the day—internal dryness has an adverse effect on the eyes. Hate drinking water? Add some herbal tea or unsweetened juice to the water for flavor.

Soak two cotton pads in rose water and place them over closed eyes for 5 to 10 minutes. Rose water is very cooling and excellent for revitalizing tired eyes.

A big saboteur of the eyes is sleep deprivation. If you're used to burning the midnight oil, try winding down earlier (stay away from TV and computers!) and go to bed fifteen minutes before your usual bedtime. Gradually bring you bedtime to 11 p.m. or, ideally, 10 p.m. Good sleep is essential to your health and invaluable to your eyes!

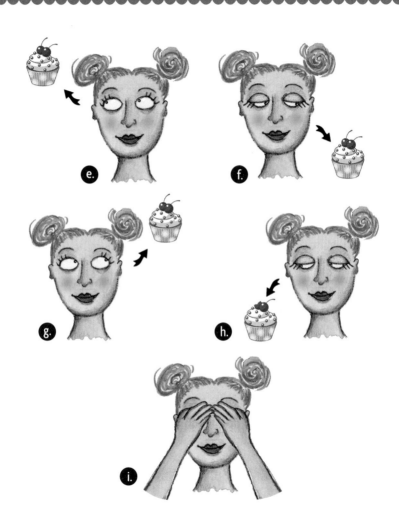

4 Without straining your eyes or moving your head—look to the upper right as far as you can at a fixed point (e.), then look to the lower left as far as you can at a fixed point (f.). Repeat 3 times, then release and blink quickly a few times.

5 Without straining your eyes or moving your head—look to the upper left at a fixed point (g.), then look to the lower right as far as you can at a fixed point (h.). Repeat 3 times, then release and blink quickly a few times.

6 Close your eyes and squeeze them as tightly as you can. Hold for a few seconds, then release. Blink quickly a few times.

7 Rub the palms of your hands together briskly, creating some heat. Cup your palms over your closed eyes. Don't bend your head. Breathe deeply while palming your eyes (i.). Hold for 30 seconds.

8 Release.

Notice how refreshed your eyes feel!

Benefits

Reduces tension in the eye muscles and reduces overall tension; strengthens and tones eye muscles; improves and preserves eyesight; relieves computer eye strain; reduces wrinkles around the eyes!

Focus Points & Tips

Keep your whole body motionless— nothing should move except your eyes; don't strain or tense up; keep your neck and shoulders relaxed; remember to retain your original posture: spine erect, hands on knees, and head straight.

Ouch   Overusing your eyes? Sitting at a computer all day? Every thirty minutes, take a break and look into the distance, and then palm your eyes (see Step 7, above.) or get up and do Standing Forward Bend Pose. Taking a minute or so to do this will reduce eyestrain and boost your energy!

Mountain with Arms Over Head Pose
(Tadasana)

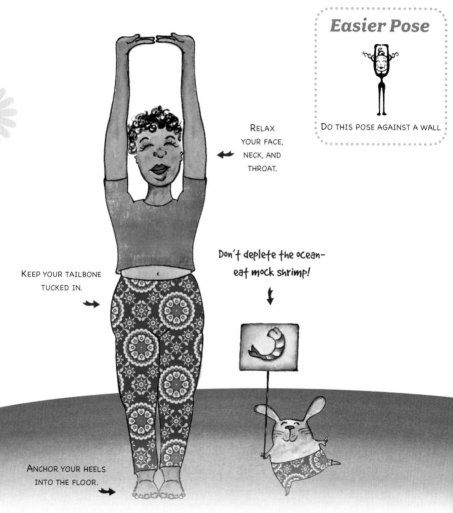

Easier Pose

DO THIS POSE AGAINST A WALL

RELAX YOUR FACE, NECK, AND THROAT.

KEEP YOUR TAILBONE TUCKED IN.

Don't deplete the ocean— eat mock shrimp!

ANCHOR YOUR HEELS INTO THE FLOOR.

Resemble a cooked shrimp?
This improves posture and elongates the spine.

3

AGELESS

1 Stand with your feet together, firmly anchored on the floor.

2 Raise your kneecaps by tightening your thighs.

3 Interlace your hands, then turn your palms down, so you are looking at the back of your hands.

4 Exhale and lift your arms to shoulder height.

5 Roll your shoulders back. Press your hands into the sky.

6 Inhale and lift arms up over your head (palms should be facing the sky).

7 Straighten your arms by pulling your elbows toward your ears.

8 Relax.

9 Switch interlacing of hands. Repeat.

Benefits

Relieves stiffness in the shoulder joints; tones and stimulates the spine and belly; relieves depression; improves posture and stability; boosts self-confidence.

Focus Points & Tips

Keep your belly soft; rolling your shoulder blades back and down and away from your ears will relax your shoulders and open your chest; press your hands toward the sky; maintain strong legs; keep your weight evenly distributed on your feet.

Ouch   Do not practice this pose for more than 30 seconds if you have low blood pressure.

Revolved Chair Pose
(Parivrtta Utkatasana)

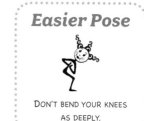

Easier Pose

DON'T BEND YOUR KNEES
AS DEEPLY.

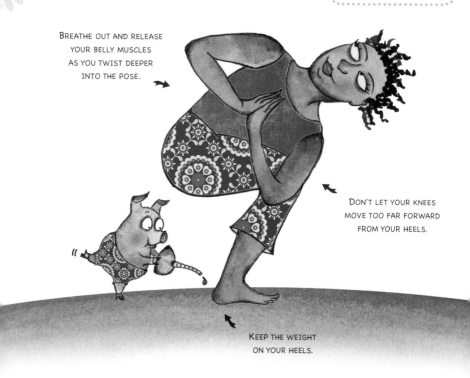

BREATHE OUT AND RELEASE
YOUR BELLY MUSCLES
AS YOU TWIST DEEPER
INTO THE POSE.

DON'T LET YOUR KNEES
MOVE TOO FAR FORWARD
FROM YOUR HEELS.

KEEP THE WEIGHT
ON YOUR HEELS.

Feel like you could use an oil change?
This brings oxygen-rich blood to all the organs of the body.

1 Stand with your feet together firmly anchored on the floor, arms at your sides.

2 Bend your knees deeply, as if you were sitting in a chair.

3 Shift your weight to your heels and squeeze your inner thighs together.

4 Raise your arms over your head, fingers reaching toward the sky.

5 Bring the palms together then lower your arms, resting your palms at the center of your chest.

6 Exhale and twist your torso to the left, bringing your right elbow to the outside of your left knee.

7 Press your right arm against your leg to deepen your twist.

8 Turn your gaze gently up.

9 Hold for 30 seconds to 1 minute.
   Repeat on the opposite side.

Benefits

Invigorating; squatting poses are very grounding and can diminish timidity; releases stagnation; increases flexibility in the spine; improves digestion; strengthens the back, thighs, abdomen, derriere; stretches the back, chest, and hips.

Focus Points & Tips

Twist deeper into the pose when you exhale; let your breath guide you and breathe into your core; lift your sit bones up toward the sky; your knees should be level with each other (don't let one ride forward); imagine the twist wringing out toxins (because it does!).

Ouch Some people with disc herniation may find relief in twists, but others may find them painful. Use caution when practicing twists, and start with standing twists. Listen to your body and let it be your guide!

Shiva Pose
(Natarajasana)

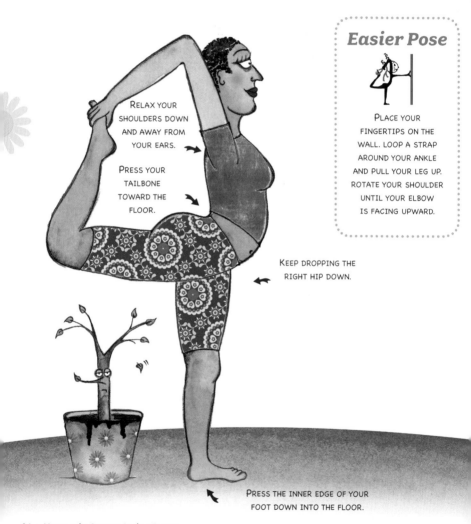

RELAX YOUR SHOULDERS DOWN AND AWAY FROM YOUR EARS.

PRESS YOUR TAILBONE TOWARD THE FLOOR.

Easier Pose

PLACE YOUR FINGERTIPS ON THE WALL. LOOP A STRAP AROUND YOUR ANKLE AND PULL YOUR LEG UP. ROTATE YOUR SHOULDER UNTIL YOUR ELBOW IS FACING UPWARD.

KEEP DROPPING THE RIGHT HIP DOWN.

PRESS THE INNER EDGE OF YOUR FOOT DOWN INTO THE FLOOR.

Are you a stick in the mud?
This will open your heart and limber your soul.

5
AGELESS

   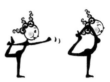

1 Stand with your feet together firmly anchored on the floor, arms at your sides.

2 Shift your weight onto your left foot.

3 Bend your right knee, reach back with your right hand, and take hold of your right foot (you can raise your left arm above you for balance).

4 Draw the right foot up and away from your body until the right thigh is parallel to the floor (try not to let your right hip come up).

5 Begin to rotate your right shoulder so your right elbow moves upward until it's pointing straight up.

6 Once you feel balanced, reach your left arm back and take hold of your right foot, using the same shoulder rotation you used with the right arm.

7 Stay in the pose for 20 to 30 seconds. Repeat on the opposite side.

Benefits

Rejuvenating and energizing; opens the chest and lungs for better breathing; strengthens the legs and ankles; improves balance; strengthens the spine and legs; stretches the shoulders and chest; encourages change and fearlessness.

Focus Points & Tips

Stand tall and keep your standing leg grounded, straight, and strong; lift your chest upward; feel your heart open.

Ouch Keep the lifted foot flexed to avoid cramping.

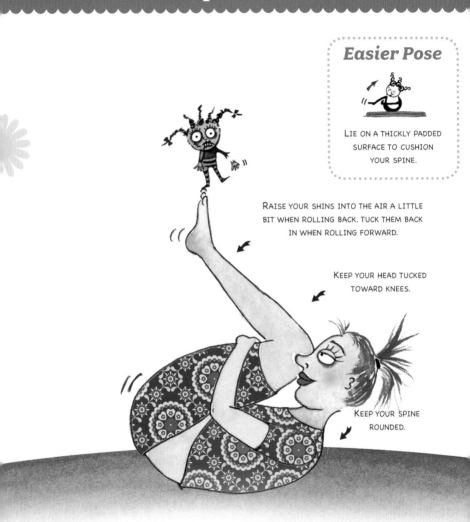

Easier Pose

LIE ON A THICKLY PADDED SURFACE TO CUSHION YOUR SPINE.

RAISE YOUR SHINS INTO THE AIR A LITTLE BIT WHEN ROLLING BACK. TUCK THEM BACK IN WHEN ROLLING FORWARD.

KEEP YOUR HEAD TUCKED TOWARD KNEES.

KEEP YOUR SPINE ROUNDED.

Walking around like a zombie?

This wakes up the body and massages the entire spine.

1   Sit on the end of a mat or blanket.

2   Bend your knees and clasp your hands right underneath them or hold on to your thighs (whichever is more comfortable).

3   Curl your head toward your knees.

4   Keeping your spine rounded, gently roll back, allowing your shins to lift up into the air (don't roll back too far onto your neck).

5   As you roll forward, tuck your shins in (this will help you gain momentum).

6   Gently roll back and forth (think of yourself as a rocking chair!) about 5 or 6 times. Feel each vertebrae getting its own personal massage.

7   Finish by lying on your back and taking a few deep breaths.

Benefits

Melts away morning stiffness and grogginess; invigorating massage to the entire spine; limbers up the spine and keeps it flexible and youthful; helps you sleep better (great for getting rid of insomnia!); relaxes the nervous system.

Focus Points & Tips

Don't roll back and forth too slowly; don't pause after you roll back, keep a nice rocking motion going.

Ouch   If you have neck problems use caution and don't perform this pose on a hard surface.

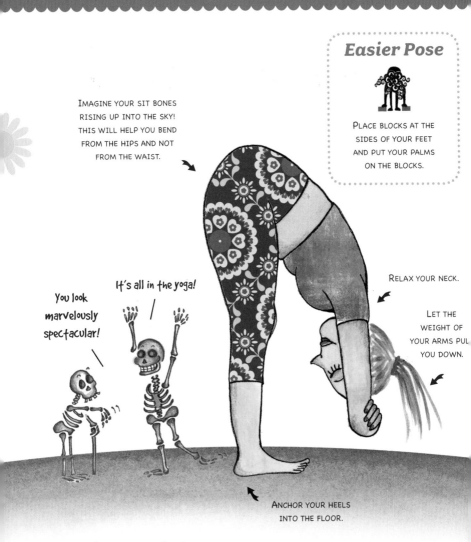

Easier Pose

PLACE BLOCKS AT THE SIDES OF YOUR FEET AND PUT YOUR PALMS ON THE BLOCKS.

IMAGINE YOUR SIT BONES RISING UP INTO THE SKY! THIS WILL HELP YOU BEND FROM THE HIPS AND NOT FROM THE WAIST.

It's all in the yoga!

You look marvelously spectacular!

RELAX YOUR NECK.

LET THE WEIGHT OF YOUR ARMS PULL YOU DOWN.

ANCHOR YOUR HEELS INTO THE FLOOR.

Feel older than Methuselah?
This softens facial muscles and reduces wrinkles.

1   Stand with your feet anchored to the floor, hip distance apart, toes spread.

2   Fold your arms and hold both elbows with your hands.

3   Inhale and lift your arms up over your head.

4   Exhale and slowly bend forward from the hips, NOT from the waist
    (imagine yourself folding over, rather than bending over).

5   Let the weight of your elbows deepen the bend.

    Hold for 30 seconds to 2 minutes.

Benefits

Calms the brain; relieves stress; relieves
mild depression and reduces anxiety;
good stretch for the hamstrings, calves,
and hips; strengthens the thighs and knees;
improves digestion.

Focus Points & Tips

Make sure your feet line up and that they
stay parallel; deepen the pose a little when
you exhale; you can bend your knees a
little and sway back and forth while doing
this pose; let go of any tension; relax into
the pose. One of the best hints is to think
of anchoring or grounding your heels down
into the floor.

Ouch   If you have disk problems, use caution. Forward bends may help the facet joints,
but they may also bring on symptoms or—worse—reinjure the area. You may
want to skip forward bends all together.

Legs-Up-the-Wall Pose
(Viparita Karani)

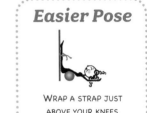

Easier Pose

WRAP A STRAP JUST
ABOVE YOUR KNEES.

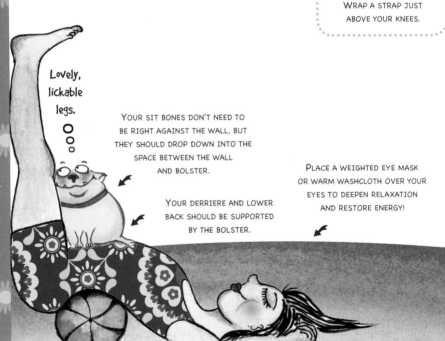

Lovely,
lickable
legs.

YOUR SIT BONES DON'T NEED TO
BE RIGHT AGAINST THE WALL, BUT
THEY SHOULD DROP DOWN INTO THE
SPACE BETWEEN THE WALL
AND BOLSTER.

PLACE A WEIGHTED EYE MASK
OR WARM WASHCLOTH OVER YOUR
EYES TO DEEPEN RELAXATION
AND RESTORE ENERGY!

YOUR DERRIERE AND LOWER
BACK SHOULD BE SUPPORTED
BY THE BOLSTER.

Do your legs resemble a Hong Kong road map?
This reduces varicose veins.

8
AGELESS

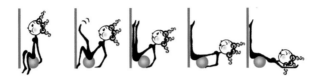

1 Place a bolster about 6 inches away from a wall, lengthwise. With the wall to your right, sit on the bolster.

2 Exhale, begin turning toward the wall, lean back (with your hands behind you for support), bend your knees toward your chest, and carefully swing first your right leg up onto the wall and then your left leg.

3 Bring your derriere as close to the wall as possible, then straighten your legs against the wall.

4 Rest your shoulders and head on the floor (your lower back should be supported by the bolster).

Note: If all of this is difficult for you, try an extra support, like a rolled-up towel and/or move the bolster or towel away from the wall slightly until you are able to get into the pose, then wiggle your way back to the wall, as close as you can get.

5 Release your hands and arms out to your sides, palms up (your upper body should form a "T" shape).

6 Close your eyes and breathe slowly and deeply.

Hold for 1 to 10 minutes.

Benefits

Blood flows from the extremities to the vital organs; calms the nerves; refreshes you; balances the endocrine system.

Focus Points & Tips

Keep legs semi-firm (enough to hold them in place); your tailbone drops to the floor; let your sternum lift toward your chin; keep your forehead and chin level; relax your entire body into the pose.

Ouch   If you have any low back or neck pain, place a rolled-up towel under your neck and/or lower back. Don't do this pose if you're menstruating.

Reverse Posture
(Viparitakarani Mudra)

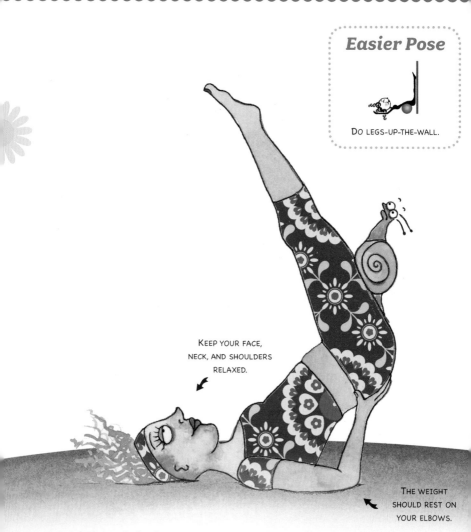

Easier Pose

DO LEGS-UP-THE-WALL.

KEEP YOUR FACE, NECK, AND SHOULDERS RELAXED.

THE WEIGHT SHOULD REST ON YOUR ELBOWS.

Feeling sluggish?

This restores vitality, prevents premature aging, and removes facial wrinkles.

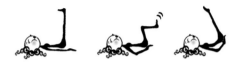

1 Lie on your back.

2 Place your hands (palms up) under your hips to help lift your hips and legs off the floor.

3 Bend your knees toward your chest and raise your legs, back, and hips off the floor (hold your hips so your body is supported on your elbows).

4 Straighten your legs and point your toes.

5 Close your eyes and breathe slowly and deeply from the abdomen.

Hold for a few seconds to 2 minutes (try to build up to 10 minutes).

Benefits

This posture is known as the restorer of youth and vitality; invigorates the entire body—keeping the glands, organs, and skin youthful; diminishes wrinkles; relieves painful periods and physical or mental discomfort during menopause; beneficial for people who have low blood pressure.

Focus Points & Tips

Your hips should rest gently on your open hands; make sure your legs are straight and your toes are pointed slightly, but keep the muscles of the feet, legs, and hips relaxed.

Ouch   Do not do this pose if you have high blood pressure.

Joy

When you're around negative, grumpy people you can feel the energy drain out of yourself as if you had a hole in your shoe! Luckily, the opposite is also true— happy, joyful people lift your spirit and brighten your life.

One of the most powerful ways to manifest joy in your life is through yoga. Yoga teaches that joy is always present and available. No matter what is currently going on in life, you only need to look into your own heart to find it.

Every aspect of yoga encourages a joyful state of being: So yoga can improve your outlook and attitude toward life. It helps keep you grounded and feel connected to the rest of the world; it encourages you to take care of yourself, accept yourself, and love yourself; and it connects you to your inner being—your Divine self.

The next time you're feeling down, try this: Sit quietly in a yoga pose (Salutation, for example). Focus on your heart and go inward. Fill your heart with loving-kindness and gratitude. Let go of stress, anxiety, toxic thoughts, and grudges. Your whole body will be tingling with joy from head to toe in no time!

Cobra Pose
(Bhujangasana)

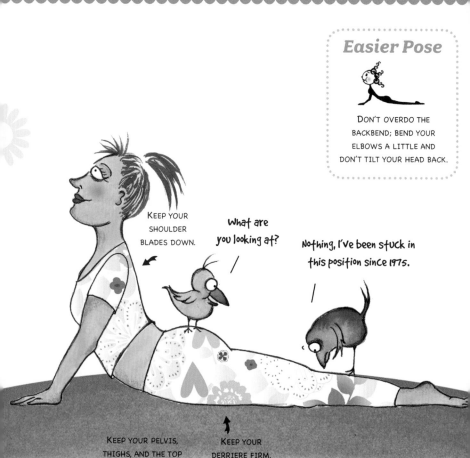

Easier Pose

DON'T OVERDO THE BACKBEND; BEND YOUR ELBOWS A LITTLE AND DON'T TILT YOUR HEAD BACK.

KEEP YOUR SHOULDER BLADES DOWN.

What are you looking at?

Nothing, I've been stuck in this position since 1975.

KEEP YOUR PELVIS, THIGHS, AND THE TOP OF YOUR FEET ANCHORED FIRMLY INTO THE FLOOR.

KEEP YOUR DERRIERE FIRM, BUT NOT TENSE.

Bent out of shape?
This baby backbend compensates for all those long hours hunched over a computer.

1
JOY

1. Lie on your belly and place the palms of your hands on the floor directly under your shoulders and close to your body.

2. Rest your forehead on the floor and place your heels and toes together.

3. Inhale and lift your forehead, then chin, then shoulders, then chest off the floor.

4. Continue curling your spine up to bring your chest off the floor. Mainly lift with the back and neck muscles; don't use the strength of your arms to lift your upper body off the floor.

5. Press your hands into the floor and slowly straighten your arms to help lift your upper body off the floor a little bit more.

6. Tilt your head back slightly and look upward.

Hold for 5 to 10 breaths.

Benefits

Strengthens the spine and back muscles; firms the derriere; relieve stress and fatigue; soothes sciatica; invigorates organs; opens the chest; improves breathing; alleviates depression.

Focus Points & Tips

Don't overdo the backbend; keep your chest moving forward and upward, so you don't strain your back; keep the image of your spine—long and strong—in your mind.

Ouch   Use caution if you have issues with your back or wrists, are pregnant or have a headache.

Seated Crossed-Leg Twist
(Parivrtta Siddhasana)

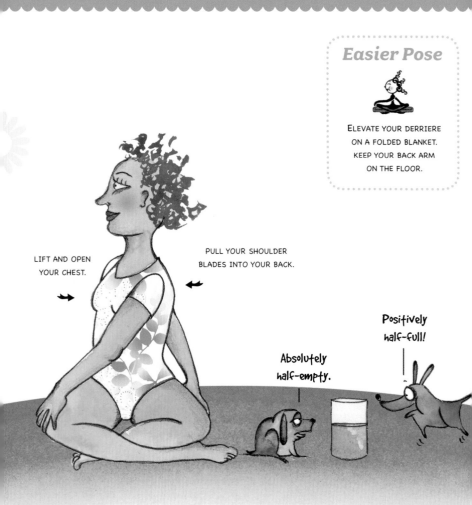

Easier Pose

ELEVATE YOUR DERRIERE
ON A FOLDED BLANKET.
KEEP YOUR BACK ARM
ON THE FLOOR.

LIFT AND OPEN
YOUR CHEST.

PULL YOUR SHOULDER
BLADES INTO YOUR BACK.

Absolutely
half-empty.

Positively
half-full!

Need to shift your perspective?

Twisting gives you the opportunity to see things from a different point of view.

1 Sit in a simple, comfortable, cross-legged position on the floor. Sink your sit bones into the floor.

2 Turn your torso to the right, place your left hand on to the outside of your right knee, and place your right hand behind your back on the floor or bring it around to rest on your left thigh.

3 Push down with your hands to lift your spine upward.

4 Pull your shoulder blades down and into your back and open your chest.

5 Exhale and twist your torso to the right a little bit more. As soon as you feel a stretch in your back, stop, lengthen your spine, and pull your shoulder blades down.

6 With each inhalation, lengthen your spine.

7 With each exhalation, twist a little bit more.

8 Gaze over your right shoulder.

9 Hold for 5 to 10 breaths. Cross your legs in the opposite direction and repeat on the opposite side.

Benefits

Releases the back; makes the spine more supple and flexible; tones and strengthens the muscles in the back; cleanses and tones the internal organs.

Focus Points & Tips

Your spine should be perpendicular to the floor; if you are leaning forward or back, place a block under your hands.

Ouch Some people with disc herniation may find relief in twists, but others may find them painful. Listen to your body and let it be your guide! Avoid twists like this during early pregnancy and menstruation.

Raised Arms Pose
(Tadasana Urdhva Hastasana)

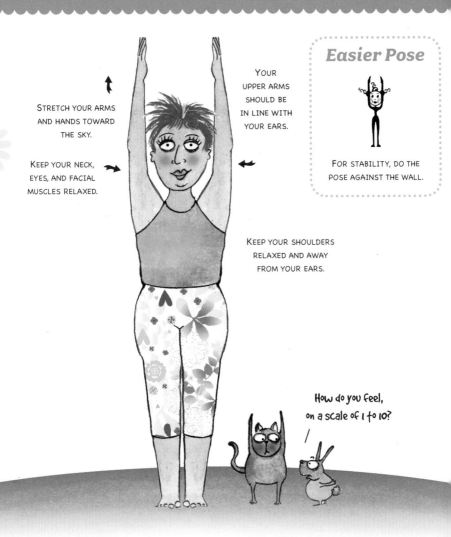

STRETCH YOUR ARMS
AND HANDS TOWARD
THE SKY.

KEEP YOUR NECK,
EYES, AND FACIAL
MUSCLES RELAXED.

YOUR
UPPER ARMS
SHOULD BE
IN LINE WITH
YOUR EARS.

KEEP YOUR SHOULDERS
RELAXED AND AWAY
FROM YOUR EARS.

Easier Pose

FOR STABILITY, DO THE
POSE AGAINST THE WALL.

How do you feel,
on a scale of 1 to 10?

Feeling gloomy?

This relieves depression and boosts self-confidence.

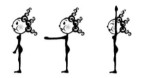

1 Stand with your feet together and firmly planted on floor (spread your toes apart and distribute your weight evenly between the heel and toes). Place your arms at your sides.

2 Exhale, stretching from the waist. Lift your arms in front of you to shoulder-level; have your palms facing each other. Relax your shoulders down and away from your ears.

3 Raise your arms over your head.

Hold for 5 to 10 breaths.

Benefits

Relieves stiff shoulders; tones the belly and spine; diminishes depression; improves posture and stability; strengthens knee joints and legs.

Focus Points & Tips

Keep your head and spine in a straight line; feel the stretch along both sides of your body; once your arms are overhead, don't pull your shoulders down quite so firmly, because it will inhibit your ability to fully reach up; continue to actively reach up (it's OK if the top of your shoulders lift slightly, just don't let them bunch up by your ears).

Ouch   Use caution if you have issues with your shoulders. Avoid this pose if you have hypertension or low blood pressure.

Extended Puppy Pose
(Uttana Shishosana)

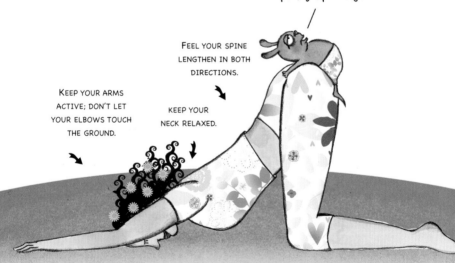

Easier Pose

PLACE YOUR HEAD ON A
BLANKET AND PLACE A
ROLLED-UP BLANKET OR
BOLSTER BETWEEN YOUR
THIGHS AND CALVES.

It's all just one big blur.

FEEL YOUR SPINE
LENGTHEN IN BOTH
DIRECTIONS.

KEEP YOUR
NECK RELAXED.

KEEP YOUR ARMS
ACTIVE; DON'T LET
YOUR ELBOWS TOUCH
THE GROUND.

Feel like a limp dishrag?
This will revitalize you and lift your mood!

4
JOY

1. Stand on your hands and knees, with your wrists directly below your shoulders and your knees directly below your hips. Your knees and feet should be hip distance apart.

2. Walk your hands forward a few inches and curl your toes under.

3. Exhale, move your derriere back toward your heels, and lengthen your spine.

4. Keep your elbows off the floor and your arms active. Press your shoulder blades into your back.

5. Lower your forehead to the floor and relax your neck.

6. Press your hands into the floor and stretch through your arms while pulling your hips back toward your heels. Keep a slight curve in your lower back.

   Hold for 10 to 15 breaths.

Benefits

Releases tension in your back and shoulders; reduces general stress and tension (when you feel overly stressed, incorporate this pose into a regular routine); great for getting rid of insomnia.

Focus Points & Tips

Concentrate on your breathing and make sure you breathe into your back. For maximum benefit, breathe in the same amount of time as you breathe out; it is important to get a good stretch in the back, and the best way is to push down with your hands and pull back with your hips at the same time, feeling the spine lengthen in both directions!

Ouch   If you have knee issues, use caution.

Fish Pose
(Matsyasana)

Easier Pose

REDUCE THE ARCH OF YOUR CHEST OR PLACE A THICKLY FOLDED BLANKET UNDER THE BACK OF YOUR HEAD.

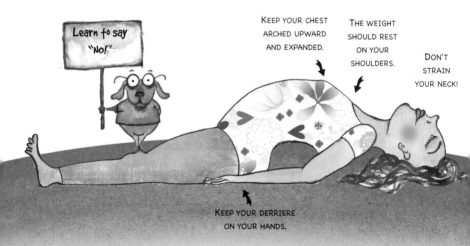

Learn to say "No!"

KEEP YOUR CHEST ARCHED UPWARD AND EXPANDED.

THE WEIGHT SHOULD REST ON YOUR SHOULDERS.

DON'T STRAIN YOUR NECK!

KEEP YOUR DERRIERE ON YOUR HANDS.

1. Lie on your back with your knees bent and feet together, flat on the floor.

2. Lift your hips off the floor a little bit and slide your hands (palms down) under your derriere, near your thighs. Lower your derriere onto your hands. Lower your legs back onto the floor.

3. With your forearms and elbows tucked close to your torso, bend your elbows and press them firmly into the floor. Use your elbows and forearms to raise your chest as high as possible off the floor.

4. Slowly drop your head back and rest the crown of your head on the floor—chin pointing toward the sky.

   Hold for 5 to 10 breaths.

Benefits

Traditional text says this is a destroyer of all diseases; stretches belly muscles and the front of the neck; stimulates the organs of the belly and throat; strengthens the muscles of the upper back and the back of the neck; improves posture; diminishes depression.

Focus Points & Tips

This backbend can be a challenge; you can support your back on a thickly rolled blanket; be sure your head rests comfortably on the floor and your throat is soft.

Ouch   Use caution if you have issues with your lower back, neck, or blood pressure (high or low).

Gate Pose
(Parighasana)

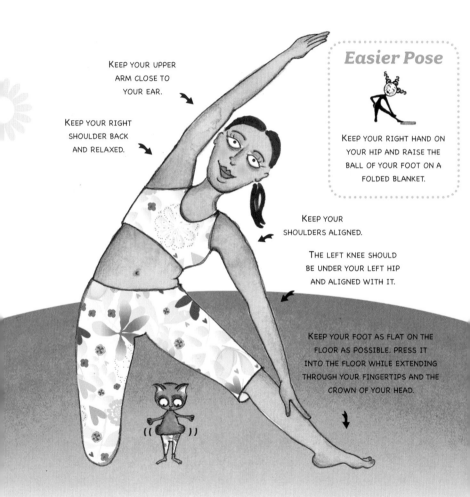

KEEP YOUR UPPER ARM CLOSE TO YOUR EAR.

KEEP YOUR RIGHT SHOULDER BACK AND RELAXED.

Easier Pose

KEEP YOUR RIGHT HAND ON YOUR HIP AND RAISE THE BALL OF YOUR FOOT ON A FOLDED BLANKET.

KEEP YOUR SHOULDERS ALIGNED.

THE LEFT KNEE SHOULD BE UNDER YOUR LEFT HIP AND ALIGNED WITH IT.

KEEP YOUR FOOT AS FLAT ON THE FLOOR AS POSSIBLE. PRESS IT INTO THE FLOOR WHILE EXTENDING THROUGH YOUR FINGERTIPS AND THE CROWN OF YOUR HEAD.

Love handles putting a damper on your joy?

This strengthens and tones all the layers of your belly muscles.

1 Kneel on the floor (a soft surface will help knees) and stretch your left foot out to the side, the left heel in line with the right knee.

2 Keep your left leg straight and strong with the knee facing the ceiling. Try to place your foot flat on the floor (if you can't, place a folded blanket under your toes until they have a firm support).

3 Place your left hand on your left thigh.

4 Tuck your tailbone in and lengthen your spine.

5 Raise your right arm, keeping your right hip over your right knee. Bend from the waist and stretch your right arm over your head, palm facing down.

6 Slide your left hand farther down on your left thigh. Feel the stretch through the entire right side, from your knee to your fingertips.

7 Look straight ahead or turn and gaze up toward the sky, keeping the back of your neck long.

Hold for 5 to 10 breaths. Repeat on the opposite side.

Benefits

Tones the belly; relieves neck and shoulder tension; improves circulation and increases the flexibility of the spine; improves breathing; great pose for people with asthma, allergies, colds, or the flu.

Focus Points & Tips

Your core/the center of your body (the abdominal muscles and those of the mid to lower back) anchors you in place, not the hand on the leg; keep your shoulders, hips, and chest facing forward throughout the pose. Find your symmetry.

Ouch   If you have issues with your knees, kneeling might be difficult or impossible, so do the pose sitting on a chair. Stretch one leg out to the side, mimicking the full pose. Perform this exercise cautiously if you suffer from knee, hip, or shoulder problems.

Revolved Head-to-Knee Pose
(Parivrtta Janu Sirsasana)

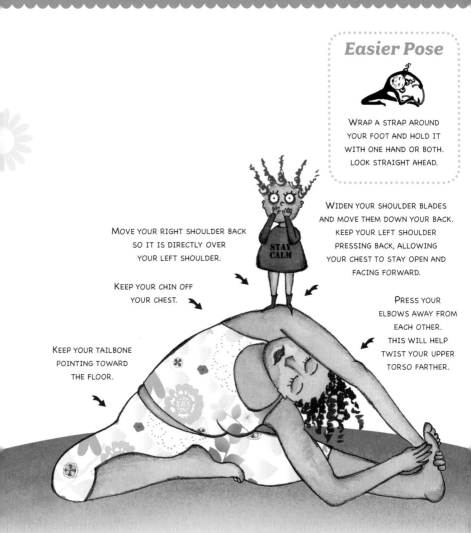

Easier Pose

WRAP A STRAP AROUND YOUR FOOT AND HOLD IT WITH ONE HAND OR BOTH. LOOK STRAIGHT AHEAD.

WIDEN YOUR SHOULDER BLADES AND MOVE THEM DOWN YOUR BACK. KEEP YOUR LEFT SHOULDER PRESSING BACK, ALLOWING YOUR CHEST TO STAY OPEN AND FACING FORWARD.

MOVE YOUR RIGHT SHOULDER BACK SO IT IS DIRECTLY OVER YOUR LEFT SHOULDER.

KEEP YOUR CHIN OFF YOUR CHEST.

PRESS YOUR ELBOWS AWAY FROM EACH OTHER. THIS WILL HELP TWIST YOUR UPPER TORSO FARTHER.

KEEP YOUR TAILBONE POINTING TOWARD THE FLOOR.

STAY CALM

1 Sit on the floor, centered on your sit bones, with your legs spread out as wide as you can (keep your spine long and aligned).

2 Bend your right knee and tuck the heel into your left groin (using your hands to gently roll the shin and top of the foot toward the floor).

3 Slide your left leg out until your legs are at a 90-degree angle—point the big toe and knee toward the sky (keep your knee slightly bent).

4 Sit up tall, lifting the outside of your ribs; line up your shoulders with your hips.

5 Exhale and start twisting a little bit toward the bent knee (concentrating the twist in your lower back).

6 Lean your torso to the left extended leg until the back of your left shoulder comes in contact with the inside of your left knee (bend your knee to meet your shoulder if you need to).

7 Place your left forearm on the floor, just inside your left leg, palm facing up. Hold the bottom of your left foot with your left hand (thumb on the top of the foot, fingers on the bottom).

(continued on page 60)

Revolved Head-to-Knee Pose

(Parivrtta Janu Sirsasana)

8   Press your right knee into the ground as you straighten your left leg (maintaining contact between your left shoulder and left knee if you can't keep your left knee bent).

9   Twist your upper body toward the sky, open your chest, and allow your right shoulder to roll back slightly.

10 Gently extend your right arm up toward the sky (keeping the rest of your body in position), lean it back slightly, and then reach your hand down to your left foot, taking hold of the outside edge.

11 Turn your head to gaze toward the sky or keep your eyes closed.

Hold for 5 to 10 breaths. Repeat on the opposite side.

Benefits

Great spine stretch; reduces mild backaches; diminishes anxiety, fatigue, headache, and insomnia; stretches the spine, shoulders, and hamstrings; improves digestion; adrenal glands, liver, and kidneys are cleansed of toxins.

Focus Points & Tips

This pose is anchored by the thighbone of the extended leg; keeping the bottom shoulder in contact with your inner knee is more important than straightening your knee completely; with each exhale, deepen the twist as you lengthen your spine; keep your belly relaxed and slightly lifted to breathe freely.

Ouch If you have knee, hip, arm, or shoulder issues, use caution. Some people with disc herniation may find relief in twists, but others may find them painful. Listen to your body and let it be your guide! Avoid twists like this during early pregnancy and menstruation.

Inverted Staff Pose
(Viparita Dandasana)

Easier Pose

REST YOUR HEAD ON A
BOLSTER OR ELEVATE YOUR
FEET ON A BLOCK.

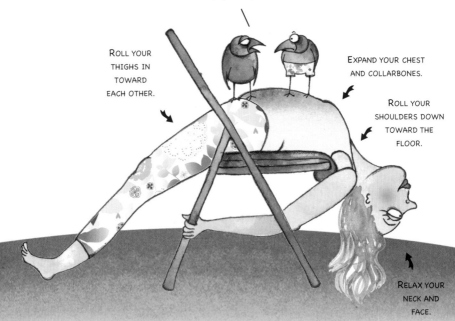

I just stayed in the nest all day and ate an entire box of mealworms.

ROLL YOUR THIGHS IN TOWARD EACH OTHER.

EXPAND YOUR CHEST AND COLLARBONES.

ROLL YOUR SHOULDERS DOWN TOWARD THE FLOOR.

RELAX YOUR NECK AND FACE.

Feel like staying under the covers all day with a box of donuts?

This relieves depression, improves circulation, and invigorates the body.

1 Place the back of a sturdy chair two feet from a wall and place a folded blanket on the chair.

2 Sit on the chair facing the wall with your legs through the back of the chair (your legs together).

3 Slide your hands down the sides of the chair and slowly lean back, supporting yourself on your elbows (your head and neck should extend past the front of chair).

4 Arch your back and rest your shoulder blades at the front edge of the seat.

5 Press your feet into the wall with strong legs.

6 Hold the back of your legs off the chair.

7 Slowly lower your head back.

Hold for 5 to 10 breaths.

Benefits

Revitalizes the central nervous system and invigorates the whole body; excellent against depression; heightens the senses; improves sitting and standing postures; opens the chest and improves breathing and circulation; tones internal organs.

Focus Points & Tips

If you feel pain in your lower back, place your feet on a block or bolster. If you have neck problems, rest your head on a bolster, press your thighs down, and stretch your legs long. You can keep your hands on the sides of the chair or the legs, whichever is more comfortable.

Ouch Avoid this pose if you have neck issues, a migraine, or a headache.

Pain

An unused and neglected body is a painful body: imbalances, inflexible spine, dry or out of alignment joints, weak and tight muscles, lack of oxygen, and stagnant lymph system are only a few of the by-products of a couch potato lifestyle. (Actually, you don't even have to be a couch potato, many people have weak and tight muscles.)

So, why not introduce a little bit of yoga into your daily life? Yoga will lubricate those dry joints, bring oxygen-rich blood to places you never knew existed, and it will elongate those tight muscles, make the spine supple, and so much more!

There are many facets to pain, and yoga addresses every single one of them with the precision of a Samurai: Yoga diminishes stress, calms painful emotions, induces relaxation, transforms thoughts, disciplines the mind to ignore pain, and increases joy.

Yoga also teaches you that the mind is a very powerful tool for healing the body, so you can transform chronic pain.

Wrist Relief

Easier Pose

ELIMINATE STEPS 4 AND 5.

I've told her a million times to get off that computer and graze in the fields with me, but she never listens.

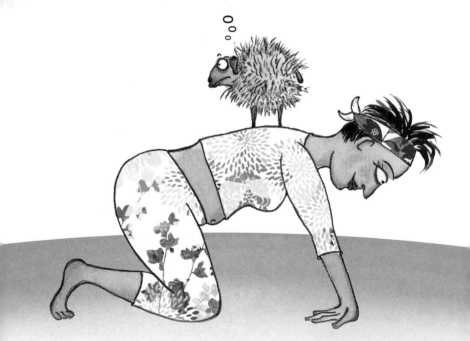

Spending long hours at the keyboard?
This relieves excessive use of hands and gives them a good stretch.

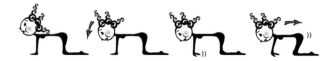

1   Kneel on all fours—arms shoulder-width apart and toes resting on the floor.

2   Place your hands on the floor, with your fingers spread out a little and facing your knees (not forward).

3   Press your palms into the floor; slowly lean back a little until you feel a good stretch. Hold for a moment, then release.

Repeat a few times.

4   Flip your hands over, so the back of your hands are on the ground (fingers still facing your knees).

5   Slowly lean back a little until you feel a good stretch. Hold for a moment, then release.

Benefits

Improves range of motion of the wrists; increase wrist flexibility and strength.

Focus Points & Tips

Keep your neck in a neutral, comfortable position (centered, not tilted forward, back, or to the side); relax your shoulders away from your ears.

Ouch   If you have issues with your wrists, use caution.

Sage Twist
(Bharadvajasana I)

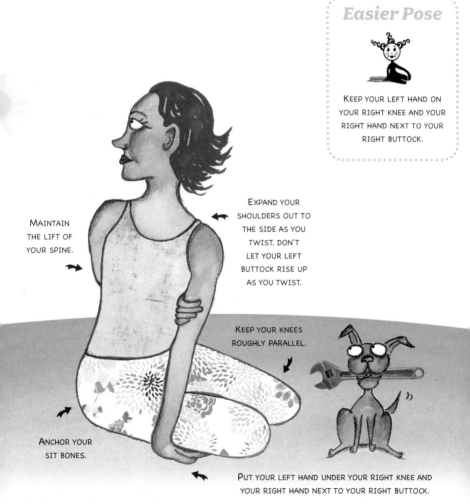

Easier Pose

KEEP YOUR LEFT HAND ON YOUR RIGHT KNEE AND YOUR RIGHT HAND NEXT TO YOUR RIGHT BUTTOCK.

MAINTAIN THE LIFT OF YOUR SPINE.

EXPAND YOUR SHOULDERS OUT TO THE SIDE AS YOU TWIST. DON'T LET YOUR LEFT BUTTOCK RISE UP AS YOU TWIST.

KEEP YOUR KNEES ROUGHLY PARALLEL.

ANCHOR YOUR SIT BONES.

PUT YOUR LEFT HAND UNDER YOUR RIGHT KNEE AND YOUR RIGHT HAND NEXT TO YOUR RIGHT BUTTOCK.

1 Kneel on the floor with your derriere resting on your heels.

2 Slowly slide your hips off your heels until you are sitting to the right of your feet.

3 Place a folded blanket under your right buttock; have the soles of your feet facing upward, your right foot resting in the sole of your left foot, and your knees parallel.

4 Exhale, twist your torso to the right, and place your left hand on the outside of your right knee.

5 Place your right hand just behind your

right buttock and use this to maintain the lift of your spine.

6 Tuck your left hand under your right knee and bring your right hand to the floor behind your back, then clasp the upper left arm with your right hand.

7 Exhale, press your shoulder blades into your back, and twist to the right a little bit more.

8 Tuck your chin in and turn your head to gaze over your right shoulder.

Hold for 5 to 10 breaths. Repeat on the opposite side.

Benefits

Relieves lower back pain and sciatica; relieves stress; improves digestion; opens the shoulders, chest, and lungs; stretches the spine, shoulders, and hips; relieves anxiety, headache, and insomnia.

Focus Points & Tips

With every exhalation, twist a little more. Don't lead the twist with your head; turn your head at the very end of the pose; continue to draw your shoulder blades deep into your back.

Ouch Some people with disc herniation may find relief in twists, but others may find them painful. Therefore, use caution when practicing twists, and start with standing twists. Listen to your body and let it be your guide!

Revolved Belly Pose
(Jathara Parivartanasana)

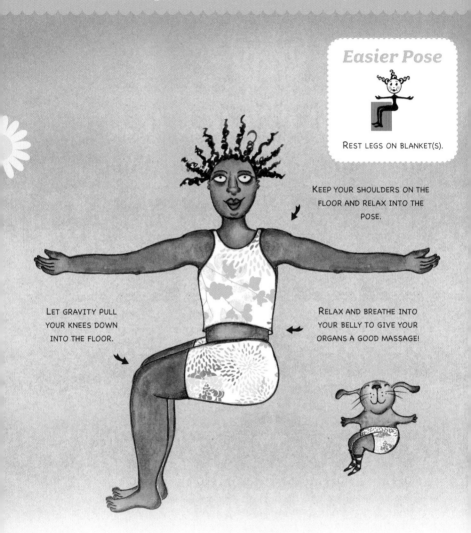

Easier Pose

REST LEGS ON BLANKET(S).

KEEP YOUR SHOULDERS ON THE FLOOR AND RELAX INTO THE POSE.

LET GRAVITY PULL YOUR KNEES DOWN INTO THE FLOOR.

RELAX AND BREATHE INTO YOUR BELLY TO GIVE YOUR ORGANS A GOOD MASSAGE!

Glued to a chair all day?

This relieves pain in the lumbar spine and releases tension from the lower back.

3
PAIN

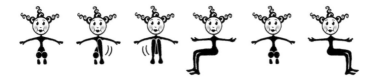

1. Lie on your back with your knees bent, feet flat on the floor, arms out to the sides with your palms facing down and hands relaxed (your upper body should form a "T").

2. Bring your knees, one at a time, toward your chest.

3. Exhale and lower your knees to the right side.

4. Stretch your arms out to the sides to move your shoulder blades away from your spine. Turn your palms to face the sky. Optional: Gently turn your head to the left and look at your hand.

5. Hold for 6 to 10 breaths.

6. Then lift your left knee up, moving it to the left side. When you start to feel your right leg lifting off the floor, bring both legs to the left side. Repeat steps 4 and 5.

Benefits

Releases tension in the spine, hips, and shoulders; very relaxing; massages internal organs; promotes better circulation; reduces stiffness in the hips.

Focus Points & Tips

If you feel stiff, slowly roll from side to side, don't hold the pose on each side; keep your head in a neutral position; sink your torso and arms into the floor; twist from the waist down; excellent pose to sprinkle throughout your practice to relieve minor aches and discomfort in the lumbar spine.

Ouch Use caution if you have chronic injury to the knees, hips, or back.

Neck Release

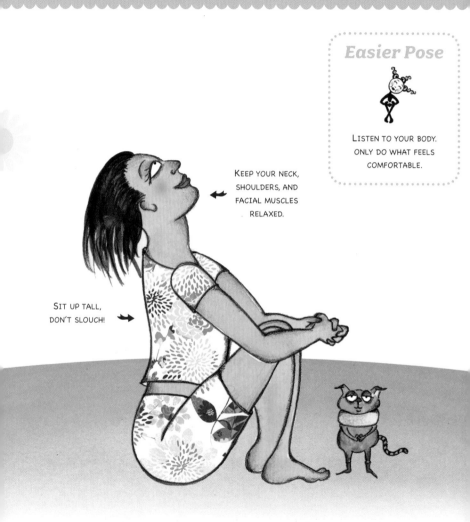

Easier Pose

LISTEN TO YOUR BODY.
ONLY DO WHAT FEELS
COMFORTABLE.

KEEP YOUR NECK,
SHOULDERS, AND
FACIAL MUSCLES
RELAXED.

SIT UP TALL,
DON'T SLOUCH!

Pain in the neck?

This decreases neck pain, stiffness, and inflammation.

Begin each of the following exercises with your neck in a neutral position (head centered and not tilted forward, back, or to the side).

1 Sit on the floor with your legs crossed, hug your knees to your chest, and distribute your weight evenly on your sit bones.

2 Tuck your chin in and gently lower your head (attempting to touch your chin to your chest). Hold for a moment.

3 Gently lower your head backward as far as you can. Hold for a moment.

   Repeat steps 2 and 3 a few times.

4 Slowly lower your right ear to your right shoulder as far as you can. Hold for a moment.

5 Slowly lower your left ear toward your left shoulder. Hold for a moment, then raise your head back to center.

   Repeat steps 4 and 5 a few times.

6 Turn your head to the right as far as you can (try to bring your chin to your shoulder). Hold for a moment, then return to center.

7 Turn your head to the left as far as you can. Hold for a moment, then return to center.

   Repeat steps 6 and 7 a few times.

Benefits

Releases tension and strain in the neck; increases range of motion; improves flexibility; improves quality of sleep; prevents headaches.

Focus Points & Tips

Do the exercises slowly and consciously; it's very important to breathe while doing neck stretches; keep your spine straight and your body relaxed.

Ouch Do exercises smoothly and slowly. Don't overdo it. Stop if you feel pain.

Knees-to-Chest Pose
(Apanasana)

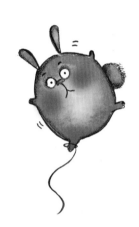

Easier Pose

REST YOUR HEAD ON
A FOLDED BLANKET.

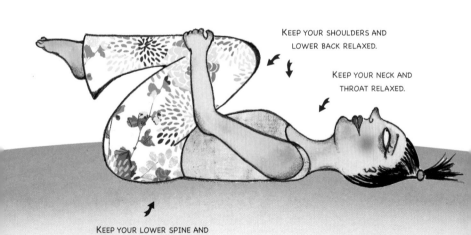

KEEP YOUR SHOULDERS AND
LOWER BACK RELAXED.

KEEP YOUR NECK AND
THROAT RELAXED.

KEEP YOUR LOWER SPINE AND
TAILBONE ON THE FLOOR.

Feel like a balloon that's about to burst?
This is excellent for relieving gas and bloating.

5
PAIN

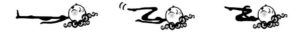

1 Lie on the floor with your feet together, legs straight, arms at your sides, and head in a comfortable position.

2 Inhale and slowly bring your knees toward your chest.

3 Exhale and, with the help of both hands, pull your knees as close as possible to your chest. Then release the hold a little bit.

4 Gently rock from side to side for 30 seconds. Or raise and lower your knees gently and slowly: Inhale and bring your knees in, then exhale and let them move away from your body.

Benefits

Releases tension in the lower back; excellent for addressing IBS (irritable bowel syndrome); relieves PMS; aids digestion and constipation; great massage to the lower back; soothing counterpose to back bends and spinal twists.

Focus Points & Tips

Keep your lower spine all the way down to the tailbone in contact with the floor; release your shoulder blades down, and broaden your chest out.

Ouch   Helps relieve back pain during pregnancy, but don't overdo it—hug your knees gently. As your belly grows, widen your knees to allow room for your belly.

Cat Pose
(Bidalasana)

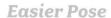
Easier Pose

PLACE A FOLDED BLANKET
UNDER YOUR KNEES.

PRESS THE MIDDLE OF
YOUR BACK TOWARD THE
CEILING, ROUNDING YOUR
SPINE UPWARD.

KEEP YOUR
SHOULDERS
DIRECTLY ABOVE
YOUR HANDS.

KEEP YOUR HIPS
DIRECTLY ABOVE
YOUR KNEES.

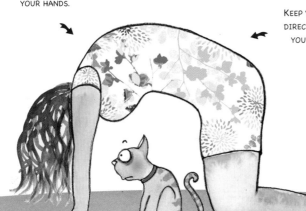

Holding tension in your body?
This is an excellent neck, torso, and back stretch.

6
PAIN

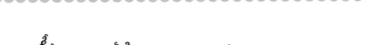
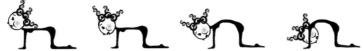

1 Start on your hands and knees, with your hands directly beneath your shoulders and your knees directly below your hips. Keep your knees and hands hip distance apart, fingers spread out, and middle finger pointing forward.

2 Keep your head in neutral position and look at the floor.

3 Exhale, press downward with your hands, and round your spine up toward the sky (like a cat arching its back);

pull your belly muscles into your spine, tuck your tailbone under, and gently squeeze your derriere.

4 Slowly curl your head inward. Gaze at your belly button.

5 Inhale and come back to neutral position.

Repeat 5 to 10 times. (This is excellent to pair with the Cow Face Pose.)

Benefits

Relieves tension in the lower back; improves digestion; breathes new life into the spine and internal organs; massages the spine and keeps it supple.

Focus Points & Tips

Keep your awareness on your back and neck; press your hands firmly into the floor to maintain the lift of the spine; use your hands and knees as support and do not arch your back more than is comfortable.

Ouch If you have issues with your neck, keep your head in line with your torso.

Cow Face Pose
(Gomukhasana)

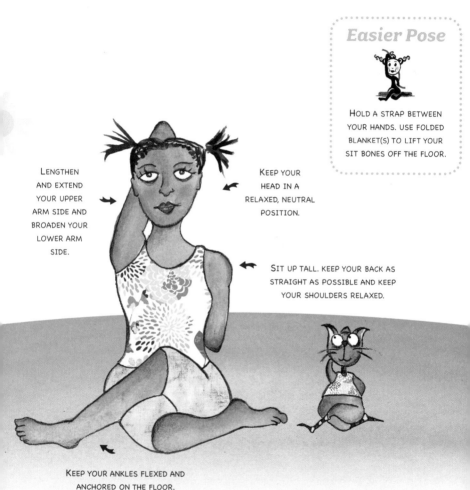

Easier Pose

HOLD A STRAP BETWEEN
YOUR HANDS. USE FOLDED
BLANKET(S) TO LIFT YOUR
SIT BONES OFF THE FLOOR.

LENGTHEN
AND EXTEND
YOUR UPPER
ARM SIDE AND
BROADEN YOUR
LOWER ARM
SIDE.

KEEP YOUR
HEAD IN A
RELAXED, NEUTRAL
POSITION.

SIT UP TALL. KEEP YOUR BACK AS
STRAIGHT AS POSSIBLE AND KEEP
YOUR SHOULDERS RELAXED.

KEEP YOUR ANKLES FLEXED AND
ANCHORED ON THE FLOOR.

Stiff hips?
This deeply stretches and loosens tight hips.

7
PAIN

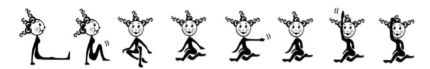

1. Sit on the floor with your legs out in front of you; bend your knees until your feet are flat on the floor.

2. Slide your right foot under your left leg until you reach your left hip.

3. Cross your left leg over the right leg, stacking the left knee on top of the right knee. Keep the heels close to your body.

4. Place the left foot on the outside of the right hip.

5. Stretch your left arm out to the side and rotate the shoulder until your thumb is facing the floor. Bend the elbow and place your left hand on your back, palm facing out.

6. Stretch the right arm up to the ceiling (thumb pointing back). Bend the elbow and reach down to clasp the fingertips of your hands together behind your back. Draw both elbows toward the center.

7. Hold for 1 minute (holding longer opens the hips and shoulders more).

Repeat on the opposite side.

Benefits

Relieves pain in the hips and lower extremities; opens the chest and expands the lungs to facilitate deep breathing; relieves tight shoulders; strengthens arms, hands, fingers, and wrists.

Focus Points & Tips

If you have difficulty resting your sit bones on the floor evenly, place a folded blanket under them and support them evenly; press your shoulder blades into your back to maintain the lift of the chest; stack knees evenly—one over the other.

Ouch   If you have neck and shoulder issues or sciatica, use caution when doing this pose. If you have knee issues, keep the bottom leg straight or sit cross-legged.

Half-Dog Pose
(Ardha Svanasana)

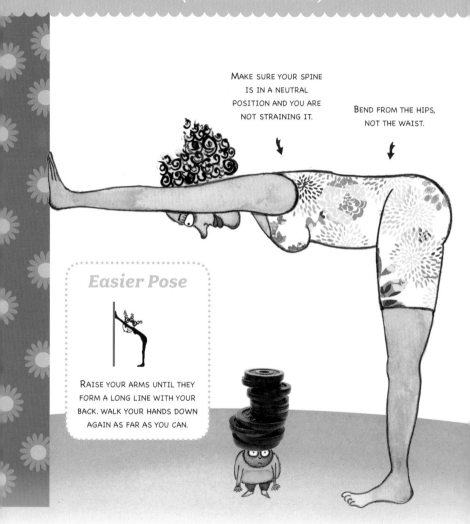

MAKE SURE YOUR SPINE IS IN A NEUTRAL POSITION AND YOU ARE NOT STRAINING IT.

BEND FROM THE HIPS, NOT THE WAIST.

Easier Pose

RAISE YOUR ARMS UNTIL THEY FORM A LONG LINE WITH YOUR BACK. WALK YOUR HANDS DOWN AGAIN AS FAR AS YOU CAN.

Feeling a bit crushed?
This eliminates compression in the back muscles.

8
PAIN

1 Stand with the palms of your hands on a wall, shoulder-width apart and level with your chest, your head and neck in line with your torso.

2 Exhale and walk your feet away from the wall, bending forward from your hips until your torso is perpendicular to the floor (you should feel a very slight curve in your lower back).

3 Press your palms firmly into the wall and push your tailbone back to elongate the spine.

4 Allow your torso to rise up a little bit when you inhale and sink a little bit when you exhale.

Hold for 10 to 15 breaths.

Benefits

Releases the shoulders, back, and hamstrings; elongates the spine; eliminates fatigue and compression in back muscles.

Focus Points & Tips

Maintain a slight curve at the lower back (if you don't have one, raise your arms up until you feel the curve).

Ouch   If the position is too stressful on your lumbar spine, bend your knees.

Hare Pose
(Sasankasana)

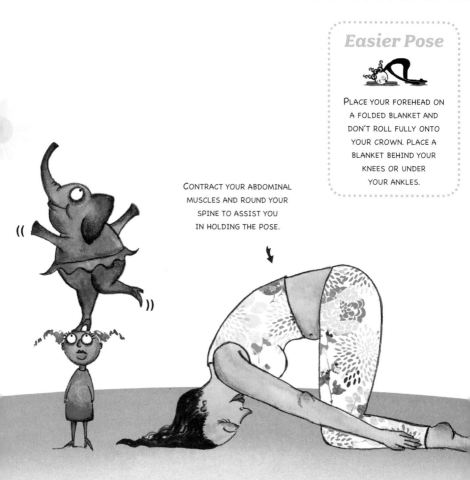

Easier Pose

PLACE YOUR FOREHEAD ON A FOLDED BLANKET AND DON'T ROLL FULLY ONTO YOUR CROWN. PLACE A BLANKET BEHIND YOUR KNEES OR UNDER YOUR ANKLES.

CONTRACT YOUR ABDOMINAL MUSCLES AND ROUND YOUR SPINE TO ASSIST YOU IN HOLDING THE POSE.

Feel like an elephant is dancing on your head?
This relieves a tension headache.

9
PAIN

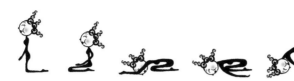

1 Kneel on the floor, with your knees together and your derriere resting on your heels.

2 Exhale, slowly bend forward from the hips, rest your chest on top of your thighs, and rest your forehead on the floor.

3 Extend your arms back, place the back of your hands on the floor beside your feet, and relax your fingers.

4 Grasp both ankles with the palms of your hands.

5 Inhale and slowly roll forward until the crown of your head is resting on the floor (use your hands and arms as support).

6 Tuck your chin in toward your chest to fully elongate your spine.

7 Continue to grasp your ankles or move your arms to the sides and keep them straight and active.

Hold for 5 to 10 breaths.

Benefits

Diminishes mental fatigue; improves the mobility and elasticity of the spine and back muscles; improves digestion; opens the hips; relieves tension in the upper back and neck; gently stretches the neck, spine, and shoulders; helps relieve colds, sinus problems, and chronic tonsillitis; good alternative pose for those not ready for headstands.

Focus Points & Tips

Concentrate on rounding your spine; pull your belly button inward; keep your chin held in toward your chest to release tense neck muscles.

Ouch   Use caution if you have neck or spine issues.

Serenity

Whether it is self-induced or external pressure, stress saturates life and often leaves people frazzled, fatigued, and disconnected from what really matters. Stress leaves people feeling lousy and looking like something the cat dragged in; it sabotages sleep and puts a strain on relationships; it destroys the neurons in the brain and increases the risk of heart disease, and more!

If there isn't a shut-off valve, and the stress keeps flowing like a river through every cell of your body, the mental and physical toll it takes won't end. You can't avoid stress—it's part of life, from never-ending bills to that loathsome, beastly boss, but you can learn to process it differently, and that's where yoga comes in! Taking a moment or two to do a calming yoga pose will calm your nerves and dissolve stress. I often find myself doing Half Shoulder Stand or Legs-Up-the-Wall Pose a few times a day, just to keep me calm and in touch with what's important in my life.

So the next time you are feeling overwhelmed and agitated, do a pose or two from this category and melt the stress away!

Vishnu's Couch Pose
(Anantasana)

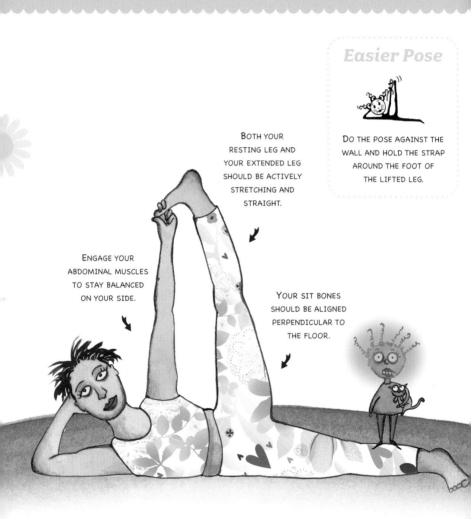

BOTH YOUR RESTING LEG AND YOUR EXTENDED LEG SHOULD BE ACTIVELY STRETCHING AND STRAIGHT.

ENGAGE YOUR ABDOMINAL MUSCLES TO STAY BALANCED ON YOUR SIDE.

YOUR SIT BONES SHOULD BE ALIGNED PERPENDICULAR TO THE FLOOR.

Easier Pose

DO THE POSE AGAINST THE WALL AND HOLD THE STRAP AROUND THE FOOT OF THE LIFTED LEG.

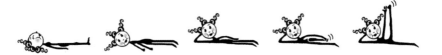

1. Lie on your back and then roll onto your right side (to maintain your balance, press your right foot into the floor).

2. Stretch your torso, lengthening your waist along the floor as you bend your right arm, and bring your right hand under your head (your arm should be aligned with your body). Rest your head in your hand.

3. Find your balance as you stay in this position for a few seconds.

4. Flex both feet, bend your left knee, and grab hold of the left big toe with the two first fingers and thumb of your left hand.

5. Exhale and extend your left arm and leg at the same time toward the sky. Straighten your leg as much as possible and point the heel toward the sky.

6. Maintain the balance on your side without rolling forward or back.

   Hold for 3 to 5 breaths. Repeat on the opposite side.

Benefits

Improves balance; stretches and tones the hamstrings and calves; improves blood circulation; alleviates the pain of leg muscle pulls; helps you focus your thoughts and start things fresh!

Focus Points & Tips

The more stability you can create by using your core muscles (in your abdomen), the easier it will be to stay balanced in the pose; flexing your feet and focusing your gaze at a spot in front of you can also help with balance; your entire body should be on the same plane (imagine you are performing this pose on a balance beam).

Ouch   If you have neck issues avoid this pose.

Downward Facing Corpse Pose
(Adho Mukha Shavasana)

Easier Pose

PLACE A FOLDED BLANKET
UNDER YOUR FOREHEAD
AND A ROLLED-UP BLANKET
UNDER YOUR FEET.

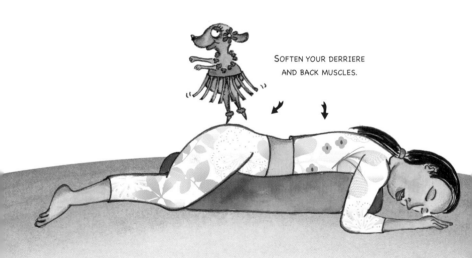

SOFTEN YOUR DERRIERE
AND BACK MUSCLES.

Could you use a permanent vacation?
This will whisk you away to a soothing state of mind.

2
SERENITY

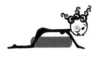 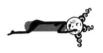

1   Place a bolster or stack of folded blankets on the floor.

2   Lie face down, with your chest and belly supported on the bolster. Drape your head, legs, and arms over the edges of the bolster and onto the floor.

3   Rest your forehead on the floor or gently turn your head to one side if this feels more comfortable.

4   Make small adjustments until you feel completely comfortable. Sink your body into the floor.

Hold for 3 minutes or more.

Benefits

Deeply soothing; melts away physical and mental tension; improves immune function; relieves tension in the neck, shoulders, and upper back.

Focus Points & Tips

Let the back of your body be as relaxed as possible; locate any tense areas in your body and release them.

Ouch   Keep your head aligned with your spine; don't turn it to one side. Use blankets and a bolster for ample support.

Fire Log Pose
(Agnistambhasana)

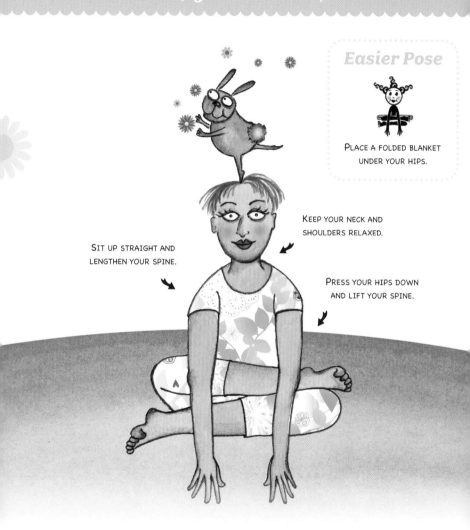

Easier Pose

PLACE A FOLDED BLANKET
UNDER YOUR HIPS.

KEEP YOUR NECK AND
SHOULDERS RELAXED.

SIT UP STRAIGHT AND
LENGTHEN YOUR SPINE.

PRESS YOUR HIPS DOWN
AND LIFT YOUR SPINE.

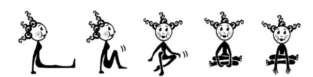

1   Sit on the floor with your weight centered on your sit bones.

2   Bend your knees and place your feet flat on the floor in front of you.

3   Roll your shoulders back and down, pressing your shoulder blades into your back.

4   Slide your left foot under your right leg and, using your hands, stack your right leg directly on top of the left, so that the right ankle dangles over the left knee (think "L" shape for each leg).

5   Press the sides of your feet down and flex your toes, to protect your knees.

6   Gently relax your knees toward the floor to open your hips.

7   Exhale and bend forward from your hips (bring your chest as close to your legs as possible without rounding your back).

8   Walk your hands forward in front of your shins or hold on to your knees.

9   Exhale and bend forward a little bit more.

Hold for 1 to 2 minutes. Repeat with the opposite leg on top.

Benefits

Stretches the hips, thighs, and groin; massages the abdominal organs; opens the hips; deeply releases taut hamstrings, lower back, and derriere.

Focus Points & Tips

Take slow, deep breaths and relax into the stretch; with each exhalation, try to reach out from your hips and lower yourself closer to your legs.

Ouch   Use caution if you have knee or lower back issues.

Half Shoulder Stand
(Ardha Sarvangasana)

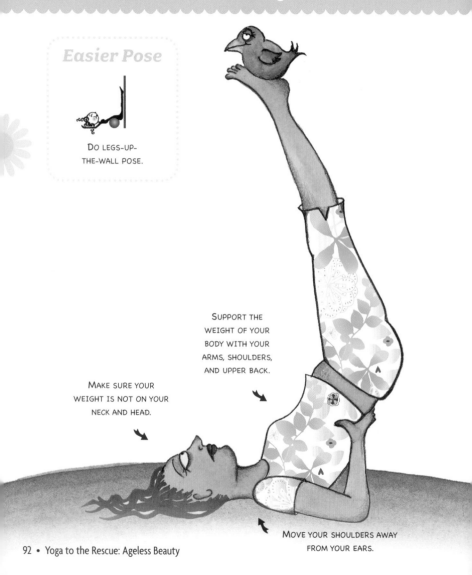

Easier Pose

DO LEGS-UP-
THE-WALL POSE.

SUPPORT THE
WEIGHT OF YOUR
BODY WITH YOUR
ARMS, SHOULDERS,
AND UPPER BACK.

MAKE SURE YOUR
WEIGHT IS NOT ON YOUR
NECK AND HEAD.

MOVE YOUR SHOULDERS AWAY
FROM YOUR EARS.

1. Lie on your back with your arms at your sides, palms facing down.

2. Exhale, bend your knees toward your forehead, and place your hands under your hips.

3. Cup your hips with your hands and start to raise your legs toward your chest, straightening them over your head.

4. Support your back with your hands, and press your elbows firmly into the floor.

5. Extend your legs up into the air. Your head, neck, shoulders, and elbows remain on the floor; your toes should be directly above your eyes.

6. Flex your feet and try to bring your elbows closer to your body, so you can roll your shoulders under a little bit more.

Hold for 5 to 10 breaths.

Benefits

Boosts lymphatic circulation; flushes toxins out of the system, diminishes cellulite; stimulates the immune system; promotes proper thyroid function; relieves stress and tension; refreshes tired legs; increases blood supply to the heart and head; improves digestion; stretches tight neck muscles; tones the legs.

Focus Points & Tips

Balance your legs over your head, so that you can relax your leg muscles; use a folded blanket under your shoulders, *not* your neck (the stiffer, less flexible your shoulders, the higher the support needs to be); this placement of the blanket protects your cervical spine; support the weight of your body with your arms, shoulders, and upper back; there should be very little or no weight on the head and neck.

Ouch   Avoid this pose in late pregnancy or if you have high blood pressure or issues with your back, neck, or shoulders.

Crocodile Pose
(Makarasana)

Easier Pose

KEEP YOUR LEGS CLOSER TOGETHER AND YOUR ELBOWS MORE FORWARD. POINT YOUR TOES STRAIGHT BACK.

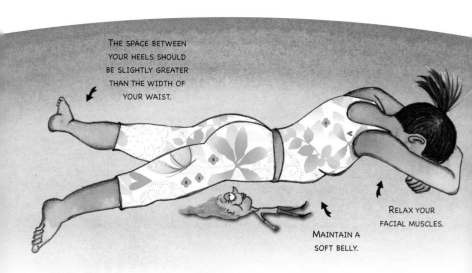

THE SPACE BETWEEN YOUR HEELS SHOULD BE SLIGHTLY GREATER THAN THE WIDTH OF YOUR WAIST.

MAINTAIN A SOFT BELLY.

RELAX YOUR FACIAL MUSCLES.

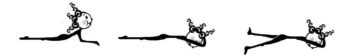

1. Lie on the floor on your belly and rest on your elbows.

2. Draw your shoulders away from your ears and bring your elbows in front of your shoulders.

3. Cross your forearms and cup your elbows in the palm of each hand, or keep your hands in loose fists.

4. Rest your forehead on your forearms.

5. Lift your chest a little bit.

6. Spread your legs a comfortable width apart and stretch them back. Point your toes outward (your feet should be at right angles to your legs).

7. Gently squeeze your derriere and press the pubic bone into the floor.

8. Tuck your chin in to elongate the back of your neck.

9. Adjust your elbows slightly forward or back until your forehead comfortably rests on your arms.

10. Close your eyes.

Stay quietly in the pose for 1 to 3 minutes and breathe from your belly.

Benefits

The perfect pose to relax the body and the mind; relieves fatigue and PMS; good for preventing or lowering high blood pressure; improves breathing—beneficial for asthma sufferers; great way to get relief from spinal problems; calms an anxious and nervous belly.

Focus Points & Tips

Stretch the whole body, from your toes to the crown of your head; feel your abdomen expanding downward with every inhalation, and feel your hips and buttocks rising upward slightly with every exhalation; your inner thighs, knees, and ankles should be in contact with the floor, as should your mouth and brow; do deep, rhythmic breathing through your nose.

Ouch Avoid this pose in your second and third trimester of pregnancy.

Salutation Pose
(Andjali Mudra)

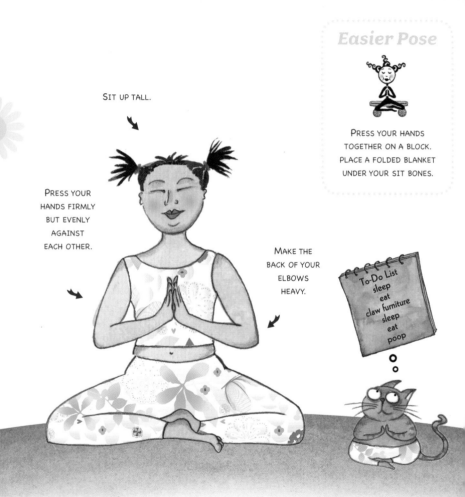

SIT UP TALL.

PRESS YOUR
HANDS FIRMLY
BUT EVENLY
AGAINST
EACH OTHER.

MAKE THE
BACK OF YOUR
ELBOWS
HEAVY.

Easier Pose

PRESS YOUR HANDS
TOGETHER ON A BLOCK.
PLACE A FOLDED BLANKET
UNDER YOUR SIT BONES.

To-Do List
sleep
eat
claw furniture
sleep
eat
poop

1 Begin by sitting on the floor with one leg in front of the other and your weight centered on your sit bones.

2 Lengthen your spine and tuck your chin in slightly.

3 Slowly put your hands together at the center of your chest (near your heart), palms together. Gently press your thumbs into your sternum.

4 Roll your shoulders back to open up the chest.

Stay quietly for 1 to 3 minutes and breathe from your belly.

Benefits

Opens the heart; reduces stress and anxiety; great stretch for the wrists; calms the brain; creates flexibility in the hands, fingers, wrists, and arms.

Focus Points & Tips

Take care not to tense your hands; the center of your hands and your thumbs should remain soft; broaden your shoulder blades to open up your chest; bring your elbows into alignment with your wrists.

Ouch Use caution if you have knee or wrist issues.

Reclining Bound Angle Pose
(Supta Baddha Konasana)

Keep a bolster and/or blankets, and a strap close by—use these props to adjust your position until you're comfortable and can settle deeply into the pose.

Easier Pose

ELEVATE YOUR HEAD AND BACK WITH A BOLSTER OR BLANKET(S), AND SUPPORT YOUR KNEES WITH ROLLED-UP BLANKETS.

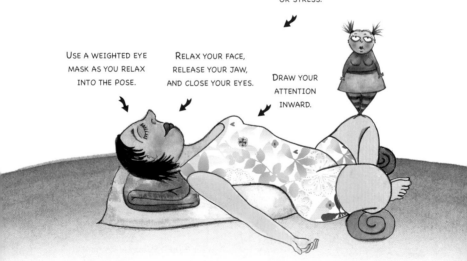

DISSOLVE ANY TENSION OR STRESS.

USE A WEIGHTED EYE MASK AS YOU RELAX INTO THE POSE.

RELAX YOUR FACE, RELEASE YOUR JAW, AND CLOSE YOUR EYES.

DRAW YOUR ATTENTION INWARD.

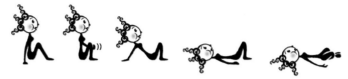

1. Sit on the floor with your knees bent and your feet together. With your hands, pull your heels close to your torso.

2. Exhale and slowly lower your back all the way to the floor, using your hands and arms to guide you. (For extra support, place a bolster or folded blanket(s) lengthwise under your upper torso and head).

3. Slowly open your knees and allow them to drop to the floor (place a rolled-up blanket under each knee if needed—the height of the blankets should be the height your knees would fall to naturally).

4. Place the soles of your feet together, and rest the outer edges of your feet on the floor (keep your heels close to your groin).

5. Use your hands to slightly rotate your thighs outward.

6. Roll your shoulders back and away from your neck. Relax your arms onto the floor, palms up.

To maximize the benefits, stay in this pose for an extended period of time, from 5 to 20 minutes.

Benefits

Restorative; improves digestion; quiets the mind; relieves PMS and menopausal symptoms, relieves mild depression; great stretch for groin and inner thighs; excellent pose for pregnant women preparing for childbirth.

Focus Points & Tips

Take time to adjust your props so that you are blissfully comfortable; listen to the messages your body is sending you; if you're holding tension, anger, or sadness in a particular part of your body, imagine it floating away; to keep the heels close to the pelvis and to relax more fully into the pose, wrap a strap around your lower torso and the soles of your feet (tighten the belt so it is snug, but not tight).

Ouch

Use caution if you have issues with your groin, knees, hips, or shoulders.

Rage-a-holic

Let's get one thing clear—anger is not bad. On the contrary, it's an important emotion that needs to be expressed. Rage (out of control, crazy anger) on the other hand *is* bad.* Not only is it unpleasant to be the recipient of someone else's rage, it is equally toxic to the one doing the raging! Over time, wanton, unchecked rage takes a toll on the heart, weakens immunity, raises blood pressure, causes headaches and digestive disorders, and more.

Restorative poses are one of the best ways to cool down rage and learn how to stay calm in the middle of a storm (a quiet body helps create a quiet mind). The next time you get passed over for a big promotion, or your boyfriend leaves you for your best friend, instead of throwing that wineglass across the room, try Crocodile or Downward Facing Corpse Pose to transcend your frustration, fury, and jealousy.

*Unexpressed rage is just as lethal. I used to think my ex-husband modeled himself after a saint or Gandhi, but in time, I realized he was just one of those individuals who thought expressing anger was bad, and he held it in, like a ticking time bomb. Holding anger in is just as hard on you physically as outward raging.

Cow Pose
(Bitilasana)

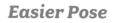

Easier Pose

KEEP YOUR HEAD IN LINE
WITH YOUR TORSO.

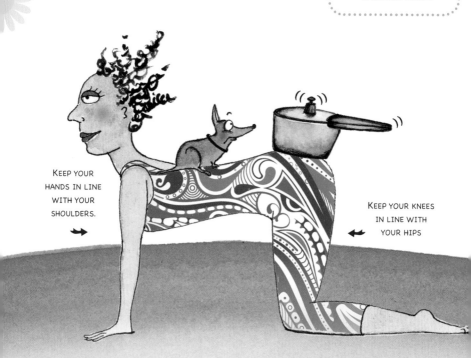

KEEP YOUR
HANDS IN LINE
WITH YOUR
SHOULDERS.

KEEP YOUR KNEES
IN LINE WITH
YOUR HIPS

Feel like a pressure cooker?
This helps blow off steam and reduces stress.

1

RAGE-A-HOLIC

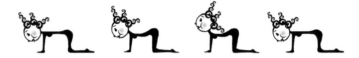

1. Begin on your hands (fingers facing forward) and knees, with your knees directly below your hips and with your hands directly below your shoulders. Your back should be flat like a tabletop! Your head should be in a neutral position and your eyes gazing down at the floor.

2. Inhale, raise your chest and sit bones toward the sky, and let your belly relax and sink toward the floor.

3. Lift your head and look straight ahead.

4. Exhale and come back to a neutral position.

   Repeat 5 to 10 times.

Benefits

Excellent stretch for the torso and back; nice massage for the spine; releases tension in the belly and groin.

Focus Points & Tips

As you bring your chest up, don't tighten your shoulders; make sure to draw your shoulders down away from your ears and let your shoulder blades expand into your chest; great to pair this with Cat Pose.

Ouch If you have neck issues, keep your head in line with your torso.

Dolphin Pose

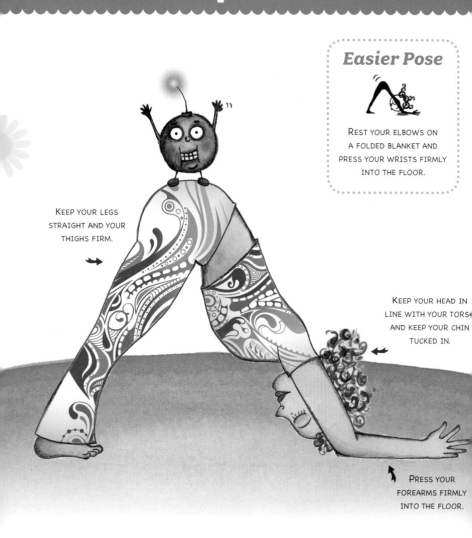

Easier Pose

REST YOUR ELBOWS ON A FOLDED BLANKET AND PRESS YOUR WRISTS FIRMLY INTO THE FLOOR.

KEEP YOUR LEGS STRAIGHT AND YOUR THIGHS FIRM.

KEEP YOUR HEAD IN LINE WITH YOUR TORSO AND KEEP YOUR CHIN TUCKED IN.

PRESS YOUR FOREARMS FIRMLY INTO THE FLOOR.

Are you a ticking time bomb?
This calms the brain and relieves stress.

2
RAGE-A-HOLIC

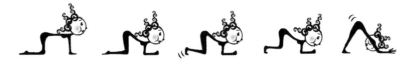

1   Begin on your hands and knees with your arms shoulder-width apart and your knees directly below your hips.

2   Place your forearms on the floor, shoulder-width apart. Make sure your elbows are lined up with your shoulders.

3   Press your palms together, fingers active (or interlace your fingers), and firmly press your forearms into the floor.

4   Curl your toes under and lift your knees off the floor (keeping them slightly bent). Raise your derriere toward the sky.

5   Slowly bring your heels down to the floor as far as you can. Your head should be in line with your torso.

Hold for 3 to 5 breaths.

Benefits

Relieves mild depression; diminishes fatigue; great for stiff and weak shoulders; especially useful for people with wrist pain; improves mental clarity and focus; helps relieve uncomfortable symptoms of menopause.

Focus Points & Tips

Don't rest your head on the floor; it should be off the floor with your neck in line with your torso; continue to lengthen your tailbone away from your pelvis, and lift the top of your sternum away from the floor.

Ouch   If you have neck or shoulder issues, keep your knees bent.

Embryo Pose
(Pindasana)

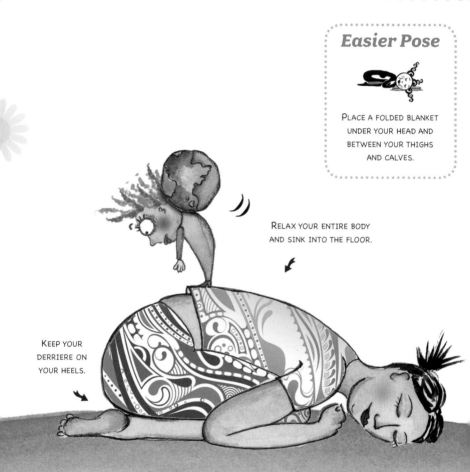

Easier Pose

PLACE A FOLDED BLANKET UNDER YOUR HEAD AND BETWEEN YOUR THIGHS AND CALVES.

RELAX YOUR ENTIRE BODY AND SINK INTO THE FLOOR.

KEEP YOUR DERRIERE ON YOUR HEELS.

Feel the weight of the world on your shoulders?
This will lighten your load and soothe your entire being!

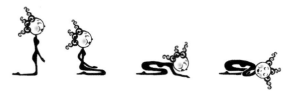

1 Kneel on the floor with your knees hip distance apart and your big toes touching.

2 Sit back on your heels.

3 Exhale and slowly lean your upper body forward, resting it on your thighs.

4 Place your forehead on the floor, then turn your head to one side (cheek resting on the floor).

5 Bend your elbows, curl your fingers slightly, and tuck your hands between your knees and chin.

Hold for 10 to 15 breaths.

Benefits

Calms the brain; relieves stress and fatigue; stretches the hips, thighs, and ankles.

Focus Points & Tips

Focus on breathing, allow your chest to rest more deeply into your body with each breath, and let go of stress and any tension in the neck.

Ouch If it's uncomfortable to turn your head, keep it straight and rest your forehead on the floor.

Half Bound Lotus Twist
(Bharadvajasana II)

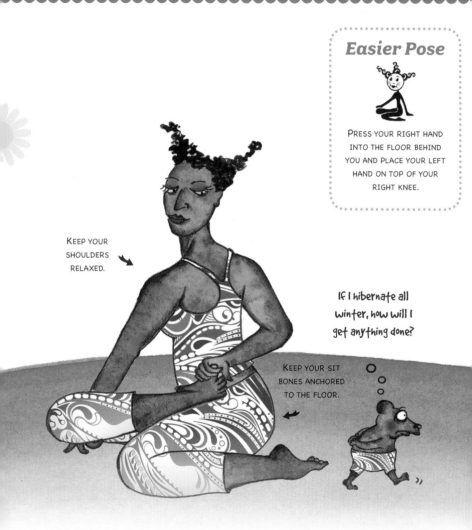

Easier Pose

PRESS YOUR RIGHT HAND INTO THE FLOOR BEHIND YOU AND PLACE YOUR LEFT HAND ON TOP OF YOUR RIGHT KNEE.

KEEP YOUR SHOULDERS RELAXED.

If I hibernate all winter, how will I get anything done?

KEEP YOUR SIT BONES ANCHORED TO THE FLOOR.

Restless? Agitated?
Twists are a great way to settle down.

4
RAGE-A-HOLIC

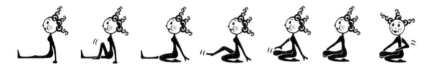

1 Sit on the floor with your legs stretched out in front of you.

2 Shift your weight onto your right buttock.

3 Bend your left knee, placing the foot next to your left thigh (the top of the foot should be on the floor with your toes pointing back).

4 Bend your right knee, lift your leg and place it on the left groin or pelvic bone (use your hands to help position your foot). Release your knee down to the floor.

5 Inhale, lift and lengthen your torso, and sink your sit bones into the floor.

6 Exhale, twist your torso to the right (keep your left buttock as close to the floor as possible).

7 Tuck your left hand under your right knee (palm facing outward).

8 Reach back with your right hand and grab the big toe of your right foot.

9 Exhale, revolve your torso a little bit more to the right, and gaze over your left shoulder.

Hold for 5 to 10 breaths. Repeat on the other opposite side.

Benefits

Stretches the spine, shoulders, and hips; relieves stress, lower back pain, neck pain, and sciatica; massages the abdominal organs and improves digestion.

Focus Points & Tips

Grounding the sacrum in all sitting positions helps to maintain and increase lower back stability. Also, in sitting twists you stabilize your hips while rotating your shoulders. In this pose (*Bharadvajasana II*), you rotate your head and shoulders in opposite directions, but your hips are stable.

Ouch

Avoid this pose if you have knee issues.

Heron Pose
(Krounchasana)

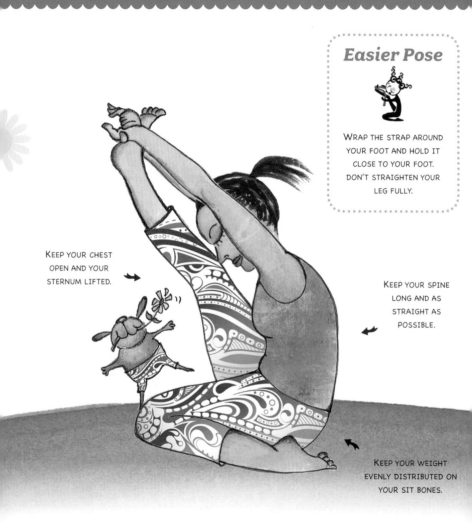

Easier Pose

WRAP THE STRAP AROUND YOUR FOOT AND HOLD IT CLOSE TO YOUR FOOT. DON'T STRAIGHTEN YOUR LEG FULLY.

KEEP YOUR CHEST OPEN AND YOUR STERNUM LIFTED.

KEEP YOUR SPINE LONG AND AS STRAIGHT AS POSSIBLE.

KEEP YOUR WEIGHT EVENLY DISTRIBUTED ON YOUR SIT BONES.

Is your life lacking tranquility?
This brings inner and outer peace.

5

RAGE-A-HOLIC

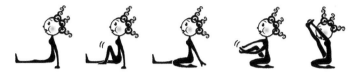

1. Sit on the floor with your legs out in front of you.

2. Bend your right knee and place your right foot next to your right hip, toes pointing straight back or slightly inward. Do not point them outward! The top of your foot should be resting on the floor.

3. Your weight should be evenly distributed on your sit bones (if necessary, place a blanket under one side of your sit bones to keep your hips level).

4. Bend your left knee and grab your foot with both hands.

5. Lean back slightly, pull your shoulder blades into your back, and slowly raise your left foot up toward the sky and as close to your chest as possible (your foot should be as high as your head, or higher).

6. Hold the arch of your foot with both hands or, if possible, grasp your right wrist with your left hand.

7. Bring your head toward your leg and rest your forehead on your knee (don't round your back).

   Hold for 5 to 10 breaths. Repeat on the other side.

Benefits

Improves posture and digestion; relieves indigestion and gastric ailments; helps people with flat feet; brings flexibility to the hips, back, and hamstrings.

Focus Points & Tips

The key to this pose is the stretch in the lifted leg. Continue to extend your straight leg to bring it toward your torso. Moving your head toward your leg is the *last* move of this pose, so don't round your spine in order to bring your head toward your leg. Instead, find the right height to elevate your sit bone underneath your straight leg. This also makes the pose safer and more beneficial; this height is often different for each side.

Ouch

If you have issues with your ankles, don't turn your lower leg outward, turn it inward and place the sole of your foot on the opposite leg, close to your groin.

Single-Leg Forward Bend
(Parsvottanasana)

Easier Pose

PLACE YOUR HANDS ON
YOUR HIPS OR HOLD YOUR
ELBOWS BEHIND YOUR
BACK. KEEP YOUR FEET
HIP-DISTANCE APART.
BEND YOUR FRONT KNEE.

LENGTHEN YOUR SPINE
AND BOTH SIDES OF
YOUR TORSO.

MAINTAIN A
LONG, RELAXED
NECK. DO NOT
OVERARCH
YOUR NECK.

KEEP YOUR HIPS
SQUARE, FACING
FORWARD, AND
WITH BOTH AT THE
SAME HEIGHT.

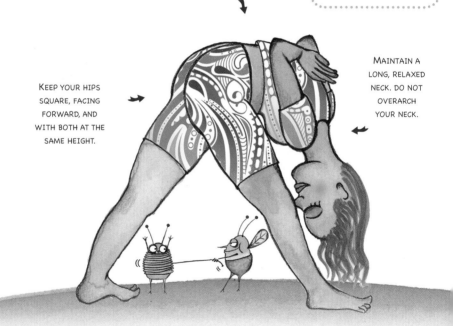

All wound up?
This will unwind you and soothe your nervous system.

6
RAGE-A-HOLIC

1. Stand with your feet together and firmly anchored on the floor.

2. Tuck your tailbone in, extend your arms out to the sides (parallel to the floor), and rotate your shoulders forward until your thumbs are facing the floor (palms facing back).

3. Bring your hands behind your back and put the palms of your hands together in prayer position (the hands should rest in the middle of your back) or grab each elbow with the opposite hand.

4. Press your hands into your back as you press your shoulder blades in (keeping your shoulders relaxed) and pull your elbows back.

5. Step your left foot back and keep your feet in line (as if you're standing on a balance beam!).

6. Turn your left foot out slightly and face your hips forward.

7. Exhale, fold forward from the hips, bring your forehead to your right knee, and place your chest on your thigh (if possible). Bring the hip of your back leg forward and the hip of your front leg backward.

Hold for 3 to 5 breaths. Repeat on the opposite leg.

Benefits

Soothes the nervous system; calms the mind and body; improves digestion; opens the heart and chest; increases flexibility of the neck, shoulders, elbows, and wrists.

Focus Points & Tips

The goal is for your spine to be aligned over the front leg as you fold forward in the next phase of the pose; try to avoid having one hip higher than the other; keep your chest as open as possible throughout the pose; keep your chin tucked in; keep the back of your neck long; keep both legs straight and strong.

Ouch

Avoid this pose if you have an injury to your hips, back, or shoulders, or if you have high blood pressure. If you have wrist issues, put your palms together, facing down.

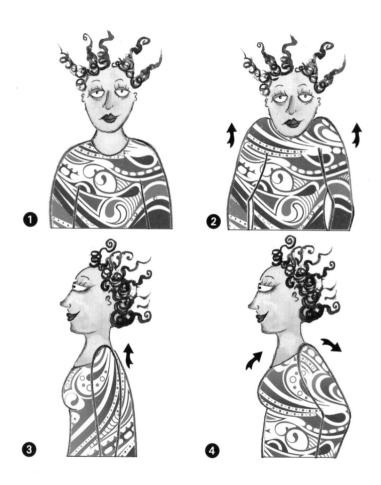

Stiff as a board?
This will loosen tight shoulders and boost your energy.

7
RAGE-A-HOLIC

Anger and stress tend to cause people to scrunch up their shoulders and hold a lot of tension there. Stop and do this quick relaxation exercise any time you feel tension building!

1   Sit or stand with your shoulders in a relaxed position and your hands at your sides. Look straight ahead, with your chin tucked in slightly.

2   Slowly lift your shoulders straight up as high as you can. Hold for a moment, then relax them completely. Repeat 5 times.

3   Slowly roll your shoulders in forward circles (visualize drawing a circle with your shoulders). Repeat 5 times.

4   Slowly roll your shoulders backward, expanding the chest as you roll (visualize drawing a circle with your shoulders). Repeat 5 times.

5   Relax your shoulders completely.

Benefits

Stretches the shoulder joints and the surrounding muscles. Reduces neck tension.

Focus Points & Tips

Maintain good posture; don't slouch.

Ouch   Do not do this exercise if you have a neck or back injury.

SuperGirl

Often, people mistakenly look for energy from external sources and imprudently seek self-confidence from others—nursing double lattes, munching on an endless array of energy bars, feeling validated when their work is complimented, and sanguine when their hairstyles or shoes get approval. This is nothing but a self-defeating, dead-end street. Quick energy fixes only lead to crashes later on; fishing for approval gives away your power to someone else . . . not a smart road to travel. Energy and confidence come from inside, and practicing yoga teaches us this.

Yoga is really good at clearing away blockages and releasing pent up energy. As a result, it can flow freely and bring you vivacity and vigor! Yoga also conserves precious energy, keeping you from expending it on fruitless activities, like worry and guilt (a real waste of energy and time!).

Like so many others, you might be carrying around so much stress and tension that your body is forced to use up your energy for support. If you learn to erase this stress and tension with the help of yoga, you will free up a boatload of energy that you can then use for the stuff you really want to do!

One Legged Garland Pose
(Eka Pada Malasana)

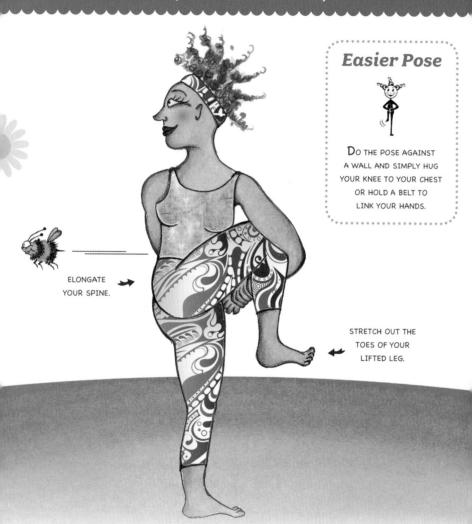

Easier Pose

Do the pose against a wall and simply hug your knee to your chest or hold a belt to link your hands.

ELONGATE YOUR SPINE.

STRETCH OUT THE TOES OF YOUR LIFTED LEG.

Have you lost your zing?

This is invigorating and will have you zipping around in no time!

1
SUPERGIRL

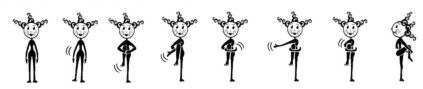

1. Stand with your feet together and your arms at your sides.

2. Shift your weight onto your left foot.

3. Bend your right knee, hugging it into your chest with the help of both hands. Take a few deep breaths and find your balance.

4. Reach your right arm forward (past the inside of your right leg) and wrap it around the raised knee (your underarm should be snug against the inside of your right knee).w

5. Rotate your arm and wrap your forearm around the outside of your right shin. Place your right hand beside your right hip.

6. Exhale, lift your chest, lengthen your spine and reach your left arm out to the side.

7. Exhale, twist your torso to the left and reach your left arm behind your back, palm facing out.

8. Grab hold of the right wrist with your left hand.

9. Turn your head and look over your right shoulder.

   Hold for 3 to 5 breaths. Repeat on the opposite side.

Benefits

Releases tension in the neck, back, and shoulders; eliminates toxins from organs and muscle tissue; opens up the shoulders; improves balance and focus.

Focus Points & Tips

Straighten your standing leg and anchor the foot strongly and evenly into the ground. Open your chest and shoulders by moving your hands away from your body (as if you are going to straighten your elbows). Increase the intensity of the pose by standing up tall.

Ouch

Some people with disc herniation may find relief in twists, but others may find them painful. Use caution when practicing twists. Listen to your body and let it be your guide!

Upward Plank Pose
(*Purvottanasana*)

Easier Pose

PLACE YOUR HANDS ON BLOCKS AND WORK WITH BENT KNEES.

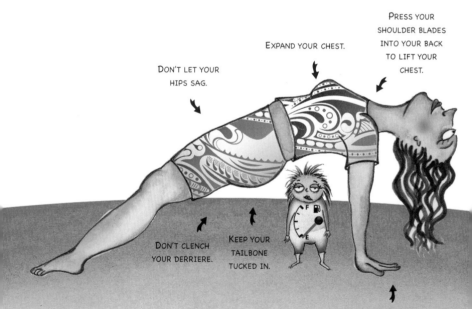

PRESS YOUR SHOULDER BLADES INTO YOUR BACK TO LIFT YOUR CHEST.

EXPAND YOUR CHEST.

DON'T LET YOUR HIPS SAG.

DON'T CLENCH YOUR DERRIERE.

KEEP YOUR TAILBONE TUCKED IN.

KEEP YOUR ARMS ACTIVE AND STRAIGHT—PALMS PRESSING FIRMLY INTO THE FLOOR.

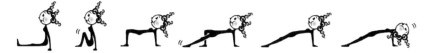

1. Center yourself on your sit bones with your legs stretched out in front of you.

2. Place the palms of your hands next to your hips (you can point your fingers toward your feet or toward the wall behind you).

3. Exhale and bend your knees until your feet are flat on the floor.

4. Lift your derriere and torso off the floor.

5. Press your arms down strongly and lift your chest until you are in a reverse tabletop position.

6. Keep your head and eyes pointing toward your chest.

7. Straighten your legs one at a time and point your toes. Press the bottom of your feet into the floor if you can.

8. As you lift your hips a little higher, engage your legs by tightening your thigh muscles, but don't squeeze your derriere!

9. If it feels comfortable (and doesn't hurt the back of your neck), gently tilt your head back, stretching your chin away from your neck. Look backward or keep your neck extended and look toward your hips.

Hold for 3 to 10 breaths.

Benefits

Tones and strengthens the whole body (especially the core); stretches arms, belly, legs, and neck; improves range of motion in the shoulders; opens and clears the chest; improves balance and posture; combats fatigue; improves endurance.

Focus Points & Tips

Align the body from the toes to the shoulders in a straight line. If it feels comfortable, drop your head all the way back. If your lower back hurts, try flexing your feet instead of pointing your toes.

Ouch

Use caution if you have wrist issues. If you have neck issues, support your head on the seat of a chair. Avoid this pose if you have carpal tunnel syndrome.

Eagle Pose
(Garudasana)

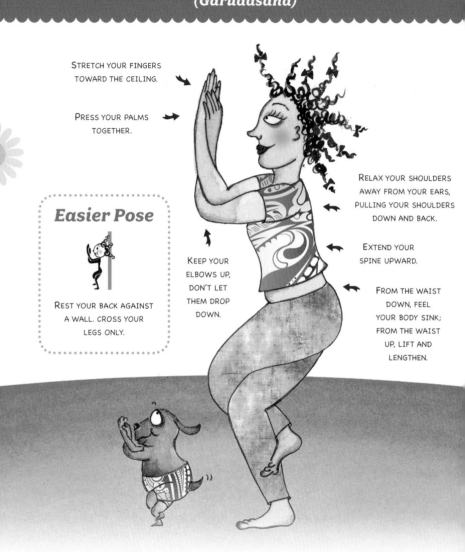

STRETCH YOUR FINGERS TOWARD THE CEILING.

PRESS YOUR PALMS TOGETHER.

RELAX YOUR SHOULDERS AWAY FROM YOUR EARS, PULLING YOUR SHOULDERS DOWN AND BACK.

EXTEND YOUR SPINE UPWARD.

KEEP YOUR ELBOWS UP, DON'T LET THEM DROP DOWN.

FROM THE WAIST DOWN, FEEL YOUR BODY SINK; FROM THE WAIST UP, LIFT AND LENGTHEN.

Easier Pose

REST YOUR BACK AGAINST A WALL. CROSS YOUR LEGS ONLY.

Want to soar like an eagle, not flap around like a pigeon?
This improves balance and concentration.

3
SUPERGIRL

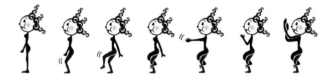

1 Stand with your feet together and firmly anchored on the floor (hip distance apart), arms at your sides.

2 Focus your gaze on something in front of you.

3 Shift your weight onto your right foot, bend your knees as if you're going to sit in a chair, then lift your left foot forward, crossing your left thigh over your right (the way you cross your legs when you're sitting in a chair).

4 Hook your left foot around your right calf.

5 Continue to balance your weight on your right foot as you stretch your arms out to the sides.

6 Slowly bring your arms forward and cross your right arm over your left; bend your elbows, bringing the palms of your hands together if you can.

7 Lift your elbows to shoulder height and extend your hands away from your face.

8 Tuck your chin toward your throat and gaze at your hands.

Hold for 3 to 5 breaths. Repeat on the opposite side.

Benefits

Gets rid of stiffness in the shoulders and relieves neck tension; increases circulation to all joints; great for people who suffer from asthma; can relieve sciatica; especially good for strengthening and toning weak legs; a great antidote to the a sedentary lifestyle.

Focus Points & Tips

Eagle Pose requires equal focus on your upper and lower body; the more you release muscle tension during your exhalations, the better your release; your weight should be evenly distributed on all parts of the foot on the floor, but don't lean forward. Take time to squeeze your inner thighs together; this will give you a solid center and more balance.

Ouch

Use caution if you have lower back, knee, or hip issues, or low blood pressure.

Crane Pose
(Bakasana)

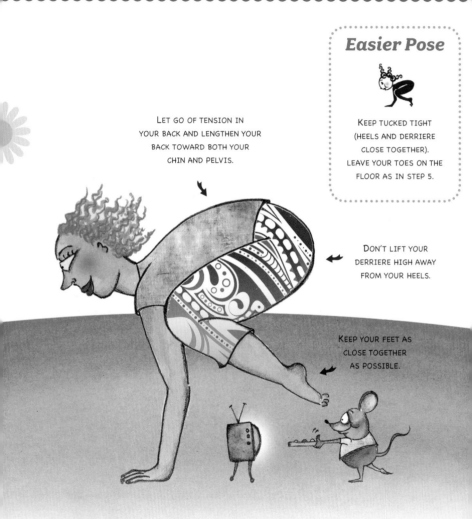

LET GO OF TENSION IN YOUR BACK AND LENGTHEN YOUR BACK TOWARD BOTH YOUR CHIN AND PELVIS.

Easier Pose

KEEP TUCKED TIGHT (HEELS AND DERRIERE CLOSE TOGETHER). LEAVE YOUR TOES ON THE FLOOR AS IN STEP 5.

DON'T LIFT YOUR DERRIERE HIGH AWAY FROM YOUR HEELS.

KEEP YOUR FEET AS CLOSE TOGETHER AS POSSIBLE.

Feel like your wrists could snap like a dry twig?
This strengthens arms and wrists.

4
SUPERGIRL

1 Squat down on the floor with your knees wide apart, and then press your forearms into your inner thighs. Take a few deep breaths to help prepare for the pose.

2 Place your hands (fingers spread out), flat on the floor in front of you, shoulder-width apart. Distribute your weight evenly on your hands.

3 Lean your torso forward and find your center of gravity.

4 With your feet close together, slowly lift up onto the balls of your feet and lean forward a little bit more (the weight of your torso should be on the back of the upper arms).

5 Exhale and lean forward more, until only your toes are touching the floor (your torso and legs should be balanced on the back of your upper arms).

6 Trust yourself and lean forward a little bit more, until your weight is on your hands; lift your toes off the floor and straighten your elbows as much as possible.

7 Keep your head in a neutral position with your eyes gazing at one spot in front of you. Hold for 10 to 30 seconds.

Benefits

Strengthens the abdominal muscles, arms, and wrists; stretches the entire length of your back; develops a sense of balance, coordination, and concentration.

Focus Points & Tips

Trust yourself and don't be afraid to lean forward; keep yourself tucked tight with your back rounded (keeping your heels and derriere close together); to protect your wrists and strengthen them, claw the floor with your fingertips; snuggle your inner thighs against the sides of your torso, your shins into your armpits, and slide your upper arms down as low onto your shins as possible.

Ouch

Use caution if you have wrist issues. Avoid this pose if you are in late stage pregnancy or suffer from carpal tunnel syndrome.

Sphinx Pose
(Salambhasana)

Easier Pose

KEEP MORE BELLY ON THE
FLOOR AND PLACE YOUR
ELBOWS IN FRONT
OF YOUR SHOULDERS.

WHILE YOUR LEGS ARE
ACTIVE, YOUR TONGUE, EYES,
AND BRAIN SHOULD
BE QUIET.

YOUR DERRIERE SHOULD BE
FIRM BUT NOT CLENCHED.

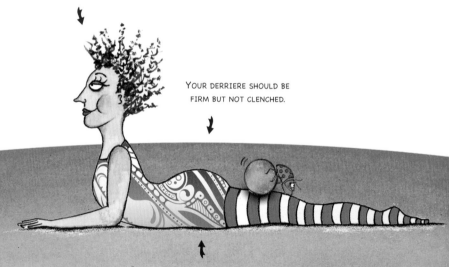

IMAGINE THAT YOUR CHEST, NECK, AND HEAD ARE
FLOATING UP TO THE SKY AND YOUR FOREARMS, PELVIS,
LEGS, AND FEET ARE SINKING INTO THE FLOOR.

Feel like Sisyphus rolling a huge boulder up a hill?
This is the ultimate fatigue buster.

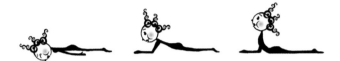

1 Lie on your belly with your legs together and the top of your feet pressing into the floor.

2 Tuck your tailbone in and rotate your outer thighs toward the floor. Reach your toes back.

3 Place your elbows under your shoulders and your forearms flat on the floor, parallel to each other.

4 With the palms facing down, spread your fingers wide and feel the weight of your upper body.

5 Press your forearms down into the floor and lift your upper torso and head away from the floor. Press your shoulder blades into your back.

6 Focus on your lower belly (below the navel). Gently draw it away from the floor.

7 Look straight ahead, and then move your eyes to look up, but take care not to compress the back of your neck or tense your throat.

Hold for 3 to 5 minutes.

Benefits

Restorative; alleviates depression; strengthens the spine and makes it more flexible; firms the derriere; improves digestion; relieves stress and opens the heart; stretches lungs, shoulders, and belly.

Focus Points & Tips

Focus on grounding your body and lengthening your spine; keep your legs and hips anchored to the floor; keep your elbows close to your sides and use your arms to lift yourself up even higher; drop your shoulders down and back and press your chest forward.

Ouch Avoid this pose if you have a back injury or a headache.

Bridge Pose
(Setu Bandha Sarvangasana)

Easier Pose

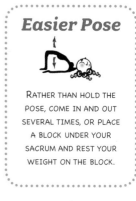

RATHER THAN HOLD THE POSE, COME IN AND OUT SEVERAL TIMES, OR PLACE A BLOCK UNDER YOUR SACRUM AND REST YOUR WEIGHT ON THE BLOCK.

DON'T LET YOUR KNEES MOVE APART.

PRESS UPWARD THROUGH YOUR THIGHS.

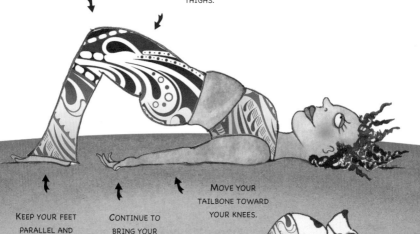

KEEP YOUR FEET PARALLEL AND FIRMLY ANCHORED TO THE FLOOR.

CONTINUE TO BRING YOUR HANDS TOWARD YOUR FEET.

MOVE YOUR TAILBONE TOWARD YOUR KNEES.

Need to reboot after a long, stressful day?
This rejuvenating backbend will supercharge your body and mind.

6
SUPERGIRL

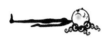

1 Lie on your back on the floor (if necessary, place a folded blanket under your shoulders to protect your neck). Keep your arms at your sides, palms facing down, aligned with your hips.

2 Bend your knees and place your feet flat on the floor, as close to your sit bones as possible (feet hip distance apart).

3 Exhale, press your feet and arms firmly into the floor, tuck your tailbone in, and lift your hips and your lower back off the floor.

4 Slowly roll onto the top of your shoulders and lift your derriere until your thighs are almost parallel to the floor (keep your knees over your heels, but push them forward, away from your hips).

5 Tuck your chin in toward your chest, press your shoulder blades into your back, and face your palms up.

Hold for 5 to 10 breaths.

Benefits

Calms the nervous system; rejuvenating; strengthens the spine and improves spinal flexibility; opens the chest; stimulates the thyroid; stretches the neck, chest, and spine; improves digestion; calms the mind and relieves mild depression; reduces backache.

Focus Points & Tips

Your weight is centered on your feet and shoulders; keep your tailbone tucked in.

Ouch Use caution if you have back issues. Avoid this pose if you have neck or knee issues and during the late stages of pregnancy.

Locust Pose
(Salambhasana)

Easier Pose

PLACE A ROLLED BLANKET UNDER YOUR STERNUM TO MAINTAIN THE LIFT OF THE CHEST, OR PLACE A ROLLED-UP BLANKET UNDER YOUR THIGHTS TO HELP LIFT YOUR LEGS.

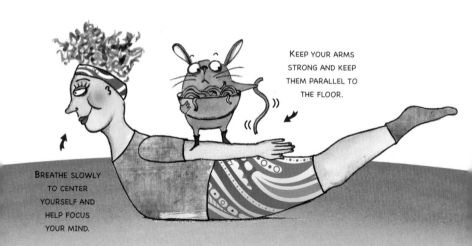

KEEP YOUR ARMS STRONG AND KEEP THEM PARALLEL TO THE FLOOR.

BREATHE SLOWLY TO CENTER YOURSELF AND HELP FOCUS YOUR MIND.

Feel like an overcooked noodle?
This strengthens the spine all the way to the derriere and eliminates fatigue.

7
SUPERGIRL

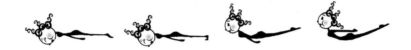

1 Lie on your belly with your arms next to your body, toes pointing back, palms facing up, and forehead resting on the floor.

2 Find your center by lightly drawing in your belly muscles, tightening your derriere, and pressing your hips firmly into the floor.

3 Press the top of your feet into the floor and tighten your thighs, lifting your knees off the floor. Roll your shoulders back.

4 At the same time, lift your upper body and legs off the floor.

5 Lift your hands off the floor and extend them back toward your feet.

6 Spread your toes and extend your feet back.

7 Gaze up, but keep your chin tucked in a little bit, to keep your neck and shoulders relaxed. You will be resting on your abdomen and lower ribs.

Hold for 3 to 5 breaths. Repeat a few times.

Benefits

Excellent back, derriere, and leg strengthener; reduces fatigue; relieves stress; improves posture; great for releasing premenstrual tension; improves digestion and elimination.

Focus Points & Tips

Actively stretch forward through the crown of your head and stretch back through the top of your toes.

Ouch   Avoid doing this pose if you have chronic back issues.

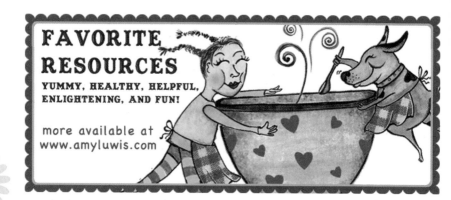

FAVORITE RESOURCES

YUMMY, HEALTHY, HELPFUL, ENLIGHTENING, AND FUN!

more available at
www.amyluwis.com

AdoptAPet.com (The nonprofit I co-founded): The world's largest nonprofit pet adoption web service, dedicated to finding loving homes for homeless animals, from dogs to horses to birds to pigs to lizards! Please adopt, don't buy.

AmyLuwis.com: Visit my website for a cornucopia of goodies—including a free downloadable bonus section of *Yoga to the Rescue: Ageless Beauty* (including material that's not in the book). You'll get indispensable tips on how to reduce stress, increase joy, and make your life a whole lot better! You'll also find healthy recipes, alternative health resources, and cool RescueGirl gifts!

Animal Liberation by Peter Singer: An excellent book that will open your eyes to the unfair, inhumane treatment of animals. It might just make you a vegetarian. We all need to tread lightly on this planet, and reading this book is a good step toward learning how.

AsianHealthSecrets.com: Want to unravel some of the mysteries of Traditional Chinese Medicine (TCM) and herbs? Then check out Letha Hadady's website and books. *Conde Nast Traveler* magazine calls her the "Martha Stewart of herbs."

The Ayurvedic Institute (www.ayurveda.com): The Ayurvedic Institute is a non-profit organization that teaches the principles and practices of Ayurveda, and it is a wonderful resource and introduction into the healing benefits of this ancient system. "Ayurveda, the science of life, has brought true health and wellness to millions of individuals throughout the ages with simple changes in daily living practices. Incorporating just a few of these proven methods into your lifestyle can bring about radical changes in your life."

BryanAspey.com: Some of the most amazingly spectacular guitar playing around. OK, I might be biased—he's also my husband....but he IS amazing!

BullyPaws.Org: An amazing rescue group where I found my lovely Isabelle. Bully Paws is committed to restoring the positive image of the pit bull breed. Due to misconceptions and stereotyping, the pit bull has found itself in the middle of controversy and debate. In many areas, tragically, the breed is banned. As a result, many pit bulls don't even get the chance to be adopted—they simply get killed. Bully Paws Pit Bull Patriots is a non-profit animal rescue group. Cooperating with local shelters, they place homeless bullies in foster homes, where the dogs are cared for until their adoption by loving families. Bully Paws takes financial responsibility for each animal during foster care and receives all funding through the generosity of private donors.

Fungi Perfecti (fungi.com): Founded by one of the world's leading mycologists. A great resource for all things mushroom—medicinal to gourmet.

The Green Grocery (www.green-grocery.co.uk/store): I have to say upfront, the creator of this fabulous organic, fair trade line is a dear friend, but even if I despised and loathed her, I'd still grab her products! Skye Connelly's salves and balms are the only thing I've found that can get rid of my severely dry and cracked "winter" hands and feet. The biggest challenge is deciding which lovely flavors to choose—Marshmallow and Lavender hand salves to Palmarosa and Orange Body Balm with Baobab Oil!

People for the Ethical Treatment of Animals (www.peta.org): The largest animal rights organization in the world. Unlike other organizations, each and every dollar they spend helps animals. "PETA focuses its attention on the four areas in which the largest numbers of animals suffer the most intensely for the longest periods of time: on factory farms, in the clothing trade, in laboratories, and in the entertainment industry."

Poses at a Glance

Ageless

| 1 | 2 | 3 | 4 | 5 | 6 | 7 | 8 | 9 |

Joy

| 1 | 2 | 3 | 4 | 5 | 6 | 7 | 8 |

Pain

| 1 | 2 | 3 | 4 | 5 | 6 | 7 | 8 | 9 |

Serenity

| 1 | 2 | 3 | 4 | 5 | 6 | 7 |

Rage-a-holic

| 1 | 2 | 3 | 4 | 5 | 6 | 7 |

SuperGirl

| 1 | 2 | 3 | 4 | 5 | 6 | 7 |

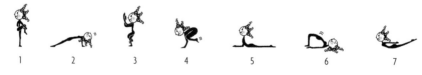

Ageless

1. Lion Pose *(Simhasana)*
2. Eye Rejuvenation
3. Mountain with Arms Over Head Pose *(Tadasana)*
4. Revolved Chair Pose *(Parivrtta Utkatasana)*
5. Shiva Pose *(Natarajasana)*
6. Spinal Roll
7. Standing Forward Bend *(Uttanasana)*
8. Legs-Up-the-Wall Pose *(Viparita Karani)*
9. Reverse Posture *(Viparitakarani Mudra)*

Joy

1. Cobra Pose *(Bhujangasana)*
2. Seated Crossed-Leg Twist *(Parivrtta Siddhasana)*
3. Raised Arms Pose *(Tadasana Urdhva Hastasana)*
4. Extended Puppy Pose *(Uttana Shishosana)*
5. Fish Pose *(Matsyasana)*
6. Gate Pose *(Parighasana)*
7. Revolved Head-to-Knee Pose *(Parivrtta Janu Sirsasana)*
8. Inverted Staff Pose *(Viparita Dandasana)*

Pain

1. Wrist Relief
2. Sage Twist *(Bharadvajasana I)*
3. Revolved Belly Pose *(Jathara Parivartanasana)*
4. Neck Release
5. Knees-to-Chest Pose *(Apanasana)*
6. Cat Pose *(Bidalasana)*
7. Cow Face Pose *(Gomukhasana)*
8. Half-Dog Pose *(Ardha Svanasana)*
9. Hare Pose (*Sasankasana)*

Serenity

1. Vishnu's Couch Pose *(Anantasana)*
2. Downward Facing Corpse Pose *(Adho Mukha Shavasana)*
3. Fire Log Pose *(Agnistambhasana)*
4. Half Shoulder Stand *(Ardha Sarvangasana)*
5. Crocodile Pose *(Makarasana)*
6. Salutation Pose*(Andjali Mudra)*
7. Reclining Bound Angle Pose *(Supta Baddha Konasana)*

Rage-a-holic

1. Cow Pose *(Bitilasana)*
2. Dolphin Pose
3. Embryo Pose *(Pindasana)*
4. Half Bound Lotus Twist *(Bharadvajasana II)*
5. Heron Pose *(Krounchasana)*
6. Single-Leg Forward Bend *(Parsvottanasana)*
7. Shoulder Relief

SuperGirl

1. One Legged Garland Pose *(Eka Pada Malasana)*
2. Upward Plank Pose *(Purvottanasana)*
3. Eagle Pose *(Garudasana)*
4. Crane Pose *(Bakasana)*
5. Sphinx Pose *(Salambhasana)*
6. Bridge Pose *(Setu Bandha Sarvangasana)*
7. Locust Pose *(Salambhasana)*

The Original RescueGirl

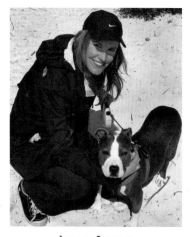

Amy Luwis is an illustrator, writer, and animal activist. She is the author of the quirky smash hit *Yoga to the Rescue: Remedies for Real Girls* and founder of RescueGirl—a company she launched to encourage women everywhere to embrace their individual beauty and to love their total package.

Tired of "up to their sacrum in seriousness" yoga books featuring perfect women in perfect poses, *Yoga to the Rescue* swaps incense and skinny-minnies for martinis and tummy rolls, without sacrificing top-notch yoga instruction; with her refreshingly human approach to yoga, Amy hopes to turn yogaphobics into yoginis, so they can discover the magical benefits of yoga.

Amy and Isabelle,
Cape San Blas, Florida

You're just as likely to see Amy rescuing a dog as doing Down Dog—in 1995 she co-founded the nonprofit AdoptAPet.com—North America's largest nonprofit pet adoption web service. AdoptAPet.com receives over 1.5 million unique visitors each month and supports over 11,000 rescues and shelters. Many animals—from dogs to cats to bunnies—find forever homes through AdoptAPet.com.

Ms. Luwis lives in Arlington, Virginia, with her astonishingly lovely husband, guitarist Bryan Aspey, and her equally lovely rescued pit bull, Isabelle.

Are you a RescueGirl? "A woman young in spirit and generous of heart who knows how to rescue herself, and who doesn't need validation because, regardless of her shape, size, hue, shoes, or status, she knows she's fabulous!"

Join the RescueGirl revolution by embracing your individual beauty and loving your total package! And get a free RescueGirl button when you do—learn more at AmyLuwis.com.